Principles of Drug Addiction Treatment: A Research-Based Guide (Third Edition)

Table of Contents

Principles of Drug Addiction Treatment: A Research-Based Guide (Third Edition)

Preface

Principles of Effective Treatment

Frequently Asked Questions

Drug Addiction Treatment in the United States

Evidence-Based Approaches to Drug Addiction Treatment

Resources

Acknowledgments

Preface

Drug addiction is a complex illness.

It is characterized by intense and, at times, uncontrollable drug craving, along with compulsive drug seeking and use that persist even in the face of devastating consequences. This update of the National Institute on Drug Abuse's *Principles of Drug Addiction Treatment* is intended to address addiction to a wide variety of drugs, including nicotine, alcohol, and illicit and prescription drugs. It is designed to serve as a resource for healthcare providers, family members, and other stakeholders trying to address the myriad problems faced by patients in need of treatment for drug abuse or addiction.

Addiction affects multiple brain circuits, including those involved in reward and motivation, learning and memory, and inhibitory control over behavior. That is why addiction is a brain disease. Some individuals are more vulnerable than others to becoming addicted, depending on the interplay between genetic makeup, age of exposure to drugs, and other environmental influences. While a person initially chooses to take drugs, over time the effects of prolonged exposure on brain functioning compromise that ability to choose, and seeking and consuming the drug become compulsive, often eluding a person's self-control or willpower.

But addiction is more than just compulsive drug taking—it can also produce far-reaching health and social consequences. For example, drug abuse and addiction increase a person's risk for a variety of other mental and physical illnesses related to a drug-abusing lifestyle or the toxic effects of the drugs themselves. Additionally, the dysfunctional behaviors that result from drug abuse can interfere with a person's normal functioning in the family, the workplace, and the broader community.

Because drug abuse and addiction have so many dimensions and disrupt so many aspects of an individual's life, treatment is not simple. Effective treatment programs typically incorporate many components, each directed to a particular aspect of the illness and its consequences. Addiction treatment must help the individual stop using drugs, maintain a drug-free lifestyle, and achieve productive functioning in the family, at work, and in society. Because addiction is a disease, most people cannot simply stop using drugs for a few days and be cured. Patients typically require long-term or repeated episodes of care to achieve the ultimate goal of sustained abstinence and recovery of their lives. Indeed, scientific research and clinical practice demonstrate the value of continuing care in treating addiction, with a variety of approaches having been tested and integrated in residential and community settings.

As we look toward the future, we will harness new research results on the influence of genetics and environment on gene function and expression (i.e., epigenetics), which are heralding the development of personalized treatment interventions. These findings will be integrated with current evidence supporting the most effective drug abuse and addiction treatments and their implementation, which are reflected in this guide.

Nora D. Volkow, M.D.
Director
National Institute on Drug Abuse

Principles of Effective Treatment

1. **Addiction is a complex but treatable disease that affects brain function and behavior.** Drugs of abuse alter the brain's structure and function, resulting in changes that persist long after drug use has ceased. This may explain why drug abusers are at risk for relapse even after long periods of abstinence and despite the potentially devastating consequences.

2. **No single treatment is appropriate for everyone.** Treatment varies depending on the type of drug and the characteristics of the patients. Matching treatment settings, interventions, and services to an individual's particular problems and needs is critical to his or her ultimate success in returning to productive functioning in the family, workplace, and society.

3. **Treatment needs to be readily available.** Because drug-addicted individuals may be uncertain about entering treatment, taking advantage of available services the moment people are ready for treatment is critical. Potential patients can be lost if treatment is not immediately available or readily accessible. As with other chronic diseases, the earlier treatment is offered in the disease process, the greater the likelihood of positive outcomes.

4. **Effective treatment attends to multiple needs of the individual, not just his or her drug abuse.** To be effective, treatment must address the individual's drug abuse and any associated medical, psychological, social, vocational, and legal problems. It is also important that treatment be appropriate to the individual's age, gender, ethnicity, and culture.

5. **Remaining in treatment for an adequate period of time is critical.** The appropriate duration for an individual depends on the type and degree of the patient's problems and needs. Research indicates that most addicted individuals need at least 3 months in treatment to significantly reduce or stop their drug use and that the best outcomes occur with longer durations of treatment. Recovery from drug addiction is a long-term process and frequently requires multiple episodes of treatment. As with other chronic illnesses, relapses to drug abuse can occur and should signal a need for treatment to be reinstated or adjusted. Because individuals often leave treatment prematurely, programs should include strategies to engage and

keep patients in treatment.

6. **Behavioral therapies—including individual, family, or group counseling—are the most commonly used forms of drug abuse treatment.** Behavioral therapies vary in their focus and may involve addressing a patient's motivation to change, providing incentives for abstinence, building skills to resist drug use, replacing drug-using activities with constructive and rewarding activities, improving problem-solving skills, and facilitating better interpersonal relationships. Also, participation in group therapy and other peer support programs during and following treatment can help maintain abstinence.

7. **Medications are an important element of treatment for many patients, especially when combined with counseling and other behavioral therapies.** For example, methadone, buprenorphine, and naltrexone (including a new long-acting formulation) are effective in helping individuals addicted to heroin or other opioids stabilize their lives and reduce their illicit drug use. Acamprosate, disulfiram, and naltrexone are medications approved for treating alcohol dependence. For persons addicted to nicotine, a nicotine replacement product (available as patches, gum, lozenges, or nasal spray) or an oral medication (such as bupropion or varenicline) can be an effective component of treatment when part of a comprehensive behavioral treatment program.

8. **An individual's treatment and services plan must be assessed continually and modified as necessary to ensure that it meets his or her changing needs.** A patient may require varying combinations of services and treatment components during the course of treatment and recovery. In addition to counseling or psychotherapy, a patient may require medication, medical services, family therapy, parenting instruction, vocational rehabilitation, and/or social and legal services. For many patients, a continuing care approach provides the best results, with the treatment intensity varying according to a person's changing needs.

9. **Many drug-addicted individuals also have other mental disorders.** Because drug abuse and addiction—both of which are mental disorders—often co-occur with other mental illnesses, patients presenting with one condition should be assessed for the other(s). And when these problems co-occur, treatment should address both (or all), including the use of medications as appropriate.

10. **Medically assisted detoxification is only the first stage of addiction treatment and by itself does little to change long-term drug abuse.** Although medically assisted detoxification can safely manage the acute physical symptoms of withdrawal and can, for some, pave the way for effective long-term addiction treatment, detoxification alone is rarely sufficient to help addicted individuals achieve long-term abstinence. Thus, patients should be encouraged to continue drug treatment following detoxification. Motivational enhancement and incentive strategies, begun at initial patient intake, can improve treatment engagement.

11. **Treatment does not need to be voluntary to be effective.** Sanctions or enticements from family, employment settings, and/or the criminal justice system can significantly increase treatment entry, retention rates, and the ultimate success of drug treatment interventions.

12. **Drug use during treatment must be monitored continuously, as lapses during treatment do occur.** Knowing their drug use is being monitored can be a powerful incentive for patients and can help them withstand urges to use drugs. Monitoring also provides an early indication of a return to drug use, signaling a possible need to adjust an individual's treatment plan to better meet his or her needs.

13. **Treatment programs should test patients for the presence of HIV/AIDS, hepatitis B and C, tuberculosis, and other infectious diseases as well as provide targeted risk-reduction counseling, linking patients to treatment if necessary.** Typically, drug abuse treatment addresses some of the drug-related behaviors that put people at risk of infectious diseases. Targeted counseling focused on reducing infectious disease risk can help patients further reduce or avoid substance-related and other high-risk behaviors. Counseling can also help those who are already infected to manage their illness. Moreover, engaging in substance abuse treatment can facilitate adherence to other medical treatments. Substance abuse treatment facilities should provide onsite, rapid HIV testing rather than referrals to offsite testing —research shows that doing so increases the likelihood that patients will be tested and receive their test results. Treatment providers should also inform patients that highly active antiretroviral therapy (HAART) has proven effective in combating HIV, including among drug-abusing populations, and help link them to HIV treatment if they test positive.

Frequently Asked Questions

> Treatment varies depending on the type of drug and the characteristics of the patient. The best programs provide a combination of therapies and other services.

Why do drug-addicted persons keep using drugs?

Nearly all addicted individuals believe at the outset that they can stop using drugs on their own, and most try to stop without treatment. Although some people are successful, many attempts result in failure to achieve long-term abstinence. Research has shown that long-term drug abuse results in changes in the brain that persist long after a person stops using drugs. These drug-induced changes in brain function can have many behavioral consequences, including an inability to exert control over the impulse to use drugs despite adverse consequences—the defining characteristic of addiction.

> Long-term drug use results in significant changes in brain function that can persist long after the individual stops using drugs.

Understanding that addiction has such a fundamental biological component may help explain the difficulty of achieving and maintaining abstinence without treatment. Psychological stress from work, family problems, psychiatric illness, pain associated with medical problems, social cues (such as meeting individuals from one's drug-using past), or environmental cues (such as encountering streets, objects, or even smells associated with drug abuse) can trigger intense cravings without the individual even being consciously aware of the triggering event. Any one of these factors can hinder attainment of sustained abstinence and make relapse more likely. Nevertheless, research indicates that active participation in treatment is an essential component for good outcomes and can benefit even the most severely addicted individuals.

What is drug addiction treatment?

Drug treatment is intended to help addicted individuals stop compulsive drug seeking and use. Treatment can occur in a variety of settings, take many different forms, and last for different lengths of time. Because drug addiction is typically a chronic disorder characterized by occasional relapses, a short-term, one-time treatment is usually not sufficient. For many, treatment is a long-term process that involves multiple interventions and regular monitoring.

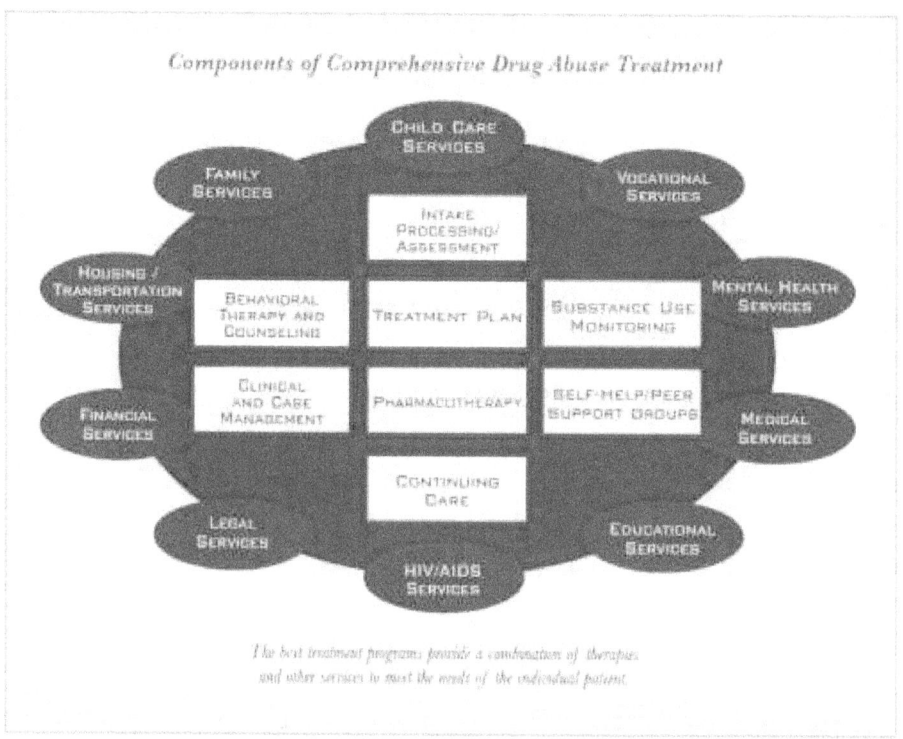

There are a variety of evidence-based approaches to treating addiction. Drug treatment can include behavioral therapy (such as cognitive-behavioral therapy or contingency management), medications, or their combination. The specific type of treatment or combination of treatments will vary depending on the patient's individual needs and, often, on the types of drugs they use.

> Drug addiction treatment can include medications, behavioral therapies, or their combination.

Treatment medications, such as methadone, buprenorphine, and naltrexone (including a new long-acting formulation), are available for individuals addicted to opioids, while nicotine preparations (patches, gum, lozenges, and nasal spray) and the medications varenicline and bupropion are available for individuals addicted to tobacco. Disulfiram, acamprosate, and naltrexone are medications available for treating alcohol dependence,[1] which commonly co-occurs with other drug addictions, including addiction to prescription medications.

Treatments for prescription drug abuse tend to be similar to those for illicit drugs that affect the same brain systems. For example, buprenorphine, used to treat heroin addiction, can also be used to treat addiction to opioid pain medications. Addiction to prescription stimulants, which affect the same brain systems as illicit stimulants like cocaine, can be treated with behavioral therapies, as there are not yet medications for treating addiction to these types of drugs.

Behavioral therapies can help motivate people to participate in drug treatment, offer strategies for coping with drug cravings, teach ways to avoid drugs and prevent relapse, and help individuals deal with relapse if it occurs. Behavioral therapies can also help people improve communication, relationship, and parenting skills, as well as family dynamics.

Many treatment programs employ both individual and group therapies. Group therapy can provide social reinforcement and help enforce behavioral contingencies that promote abstinence and a non-drug-using lifestyle. Some of the more established behavioral treatments, such as contingency management and cognitive-behavioral therapy, are also being adapted for group settings to improve efficiency and cost-effectiveness. However, particularly in adolescents, there can also be a danger of unintended harmful (or iatrogenic) effects of group treatment—sometimes group members (especially groups of highly delinquent youth) can reinforce drug use and thereby derail the purpose of the therapy. Thus, trained counselors should be aware of and monitor for such effects.

Because they work on different aspects of addiction, combinations of behavioral therapies and medications (when available) generally appear to be more effective than either approach used alone.

Finally, people who are addicted to drugs often suffer from other health (e.g., depression, HIV), occupational, legal, familial, and social problems that should be addressed concurrently. The best programs provide a combination of therapies and other services to meet an individual patient's needs. Psychoactive medications, such as antidepressants, anti-anxiety agents, mood stabilizers, and antipsychotic medications, may be critical for treatment success when patients have co-occurring mental disorders such as depression, anxiety disorders (including post-traumatic stress disorder), bipolar disorder, or schizophrenia. In addition, most people with severe addiction abuse multiple drugs and require treatment for all substances abused.

> Treatment for drug abuse and addiction is delivered in many different settings using a variety of behavioral and pharmacological approaches.

[1]Another drug, topiramate, has also shown promise in studies and is sometimes prescribed (off-label) for this purpose although it has not received FDA approval as a treatment for alcohol dependence.

How effective is drug addiction treatment?

In addition to stopping drug abuse, the goal of treatment is to return people to productive functioning in the family, workplace, and community. According to research that tracks individuals in treatment over extended periods, most people who get into and remain in treatment stop using drugs, decrease their criminal activity, and improve their occupational, social, and psychological functioning. For example, methadone treatment has been shown to increase participation in behavioral therapy and decrease both drug use and criminal behavior. However, individual treatment outcomes depend on the extent and nature of the patient's problems, the appropriateness of treatment and related services used to address those problems, and the quality of interaction between the patient and his or her treatment providers.

> Relapse rates for addiction resemble those of other chronic diseases such as diabetes, hypertension, and asthma.

Like other chronic diseases, addiction can be managed successfully. Treatment enables people to counteract addiction's powerful disruptive effects on the brain and behavior and to regain control of their lives. The chronic nature of the disease means that relapsing to drug abuse is not only possible but also likely, with symptom recurrence rates similar to those for other well-characterized chronic medical illnesses—such as diabetes, hypertension, and asthma (see figure, "Comparison of Relapse Rates Between Drug Addiction and Other Chronic Illnesses")—that also have both physiological and behavioral components.

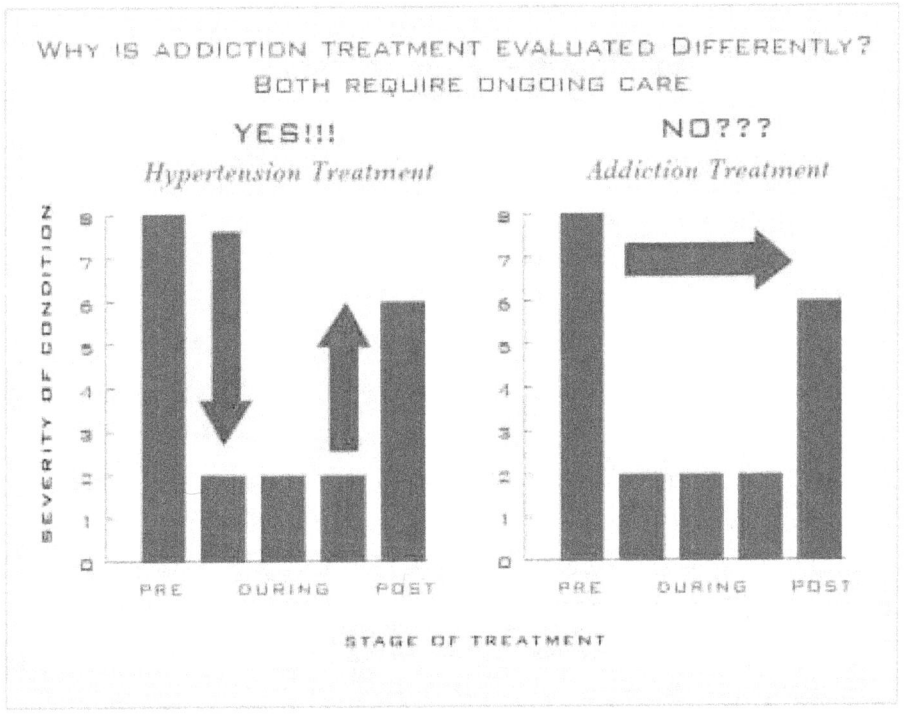

Unfortunately, when relapse occurs many deem treatment a failure. This is not the case: Successful treatment for addiction typically requires continual evaluation and modification as appropriate, similar to the approach taken for other chronic diseases. For example, when a patient is receiving active treatment for hypertension and symptoms decrease, treatment is deemed successful, even though symptoms may recur when treatment is discontinued. For the addicted individual, lapses to drug abuse do not indicate failure—rather, they signify that treatment needs to be reinstated or adjusted, or that alternate treatment is needed (see figure, "Why is Addiction Treatment Evaluated Differently?").

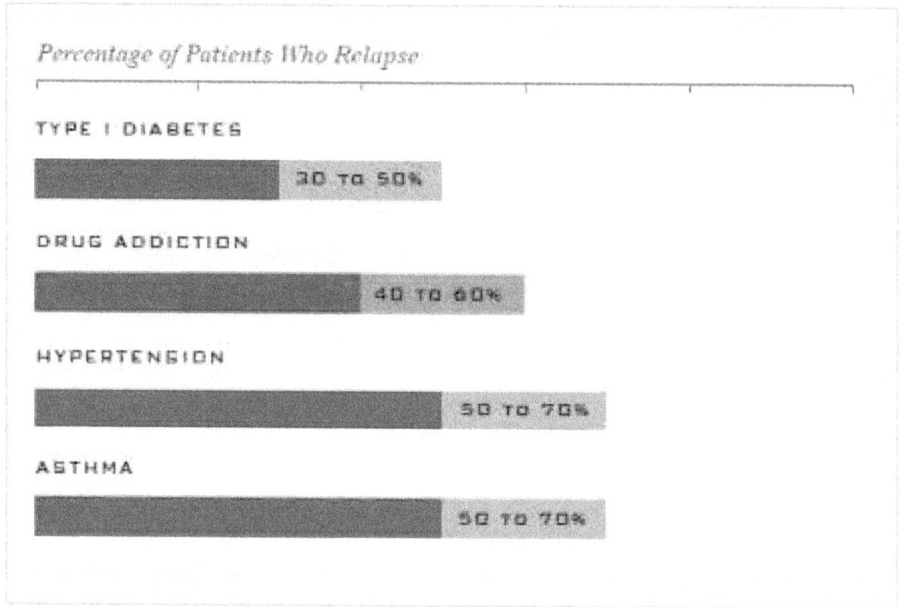

Is drug addiction treatment worth its cost?

Substance abuse costs our Nation over $600 billion annually and treatment can help reduce these costs. Drug addiction treatment has been shown to reduce associated health and social costs by far more than the cost of the treatment itself. Treatment is also much less expensive than its alternatives, such as incarcerating addicted persons. For example, the average cost for 1 full year of methadone maintenance treatment is approximately $4,700 per patient, whereas 1 full year of imprisonment costs approximately $24,000 per person.

> Drug addiction treatment reduces drug use and its associated health and social costs.

According to several conservative estimates, every dollar invested in addiction treatment programs yields a return of between $4 and $7 in reduced drug-related crime, criminal justice costs, and theft. When savings related to healthcare are included, total savings can exceed costs by a ratio of 12 to 1. Major savings to the individual and to society also stem from fewer interpersonal conflicts; greater workplace productivity; and fewer drug-related accidents, including overdoses and deaths.

How long does drug addiction treatment usually last?

Individuals progress through drug addiction treatment at various rates, so there is no predetermined length of treatment. However, research has shown unequivocally that good outcomes are contingent on adequate treatment length. Generally, for residential or outpatient treatment, participation for less than 90 days is of limited effectiveness, and treatment lasting significantly longer is recommended for maintaining positive outcomes. For methadone maintenance, 12 months is considered the minimum, and some opioid-addicted individuals continue to benefit from methadone maintenance for many years.

> Good outcomes are contingent on adequate treatment length.

Treatment dropout is one of the major problems encountered by treatment programs; therefore, motivational techniques that can keep patients engaged will also improve outcomes. By viewing addiction as a chronic disease and offering continuing care and monitoring, programs can succeed, but this will often require multiple episodes of treatment and readily readmitting patients that have relapsed.

What helps people stay in treatment?

Because successful outcomes often depend on a person's staying in treatment long enough to reap its full benefits, strategies for keeping people in treatment are critical. Whether a patient stays in treatment depends on factors associated with both the individual and the program. Individual factors related to engagement and retention typically include motivation to change drug-using behavior; degree of support from family and friends; and, frequently, pressure from the criminal justice system, child protection services, employers, or family. Within a treatment program, successful clinicians can establish a positive, therapeutic relationship with their patients. The clinician should ensure that a treatment plan is developed cooperatively with the person seeking treatment, that the plan is followed, and that treatment expectations are clearly understood. Medical, psychiatric, and social services should also be available.

> Whether a patient stays in treatment depends on factors associated with both the individual and the program.

Because some problems (such as serious medical or mental illness or criminal involvement) increase the likelihood of patients dropping out of treatment, intensive interventions may be required to retain them. After a course of intensive treatment, the provider should ensure a transition to less intensive continuing care to support and monitor individuals in their ongoing recovery.

How do we get more substance-abusing people into treatment?

It has been known for many years that the "treatment gap" is massive—that is, among those who need treatment for a substance use disorder, few receive it. In 2011, 21.6 million persons aged 12 or older needed treatment for an illicit drug or alcohol use problem, but only 2.3 million received treatment at a specialty substance abuse facility.

Reducing this gap requires a multipronged approach. Strategies include increasing access to effective treatment, achieving insurance parity (now in its earliest phase of implementation), reducing stigma, and raising awareness among both patients and healthcare professionals of the value of addiction treatment. To assist physicians in identifying treatment need in their patients and making appropriate referrals, NIDA is encouraging widespread use of screening, brief intervention, and referral to treatment (SBIRT) tools for use in primary care settings through its NIDAMED initiative. SBIRT, which evidence shows to be effective against tobacco and alcohol use—and, increasingly, against abuse of illicit and prescription drugs—has the potential not only to catch people before serious drug problems develop, but also to identify people in need of treatment and connect them with appropriate treatment providers.

How can family and friends make a difference in the life of someone needing treatment?

Family and friends can play critical roles in motivating individuals with drug problems to enter and stay in treatment. Family therapy can also be important, especially for adolescents. Involvement of a family member or significant other in an individual's treatment program can strengthen and extend treatment benefits.

Where can family members go for information on treatment options?

Trying to locate appropriate treatment for a loved one, especially finding a program tailored to an individual's particular needs, can be a difficult process. However, there are some resources to help with this process. For example, NIDA's handbook *Seeking Drug Abuse Treatment: Know What to Ask* offers guidance in finding the right treatment program. Numerous online resources can help locate a local program or provide other information, including:

- The Substance Abuse and Mental Health Services Administration (SAMHSA) maintains a Web site (www.findtreatment.samhsa.gov) that shows the location of residential, outpatient, and hospital inpatient treatment programs for drug addiction and alcoholism throughout the country. This information is also accessible by calling 1-800-662-HELP.

- The National Suicide Prevention Lifeline (1-800-273-TALK) offers more than just suicide prevention—it can also help with a host of issues, including drug and alcohol abuse, and can connect individuals with a nearby professional.

- The National Alliance on Mental Illness (www.nami.org) and Mental Health America (www.mentalhealthamerica.net) are alliances of nonprofit, self-help support organizations for patients and families dealing with a variety of mental disorders. Both have State and local affiliates throughout the country and may be especially helpful for patients with comorbid conditions.

- The American Academy of Addiction Psychiatry and the American Academy of Child and Adolescent Psychiatry each have physician locator tools posted on their Web sites at aaap.org and aacap.org, respectively.

- Faces & Voices of Recovery (facesandvoicesofrecovery.org), founded in 2001, is an advocacy organization for individuals in long-term recovery that strategizes on ways to reach out to the medical, public health, criminal justice, and other communities to promote and celebrate recovery from addiction to alcohol and other drugs.

- The Partnership at Drugfree.org (drugfree.org) is an organization that provides information and resources on teen drug use and addiction for parents, to help them prevent and intervene in their children's drug use or find treatment for a child who needs it. They offer a toll-free helpline for parents (1-855-378-4373).

- The American Society of Addiction Medicine (asam.org) is a society of physicians aimed at increasing access to addiction treatment. Their Web site has a nationwide directory of addiction medicine professionals.

- NIDA's National Drug Abuse Treatment Clinical Trials Network (drugabuse.gov/about-nida/organization/cctn/ctn) provides information for those interested in participating in a clinical trial testing a promising substance abuse intervention; or visit clinicaltrials.gov.

- NIDA's DrugPubs Research Dissemination Center

(drugpubs.drugabuse.gov) provides booklets, pamphlets, fact sheets, and other informational resources on drugs, drug abuse, and treatment.

- The National Institute on Alcohol Abuse and Alcoholism (niaaa.nih.gov) provides information on alcohol, alcohol use, and treatment of alcohol-related problems (niaaa.nih.gov/search/node/treatment).

How can the workplace play a role in substance abuse treatment?

Many workplaces sponsor Employee Assistance Programs (EAPs) that offer short-term counseling and/or assistance in linking employees with drug or alcohol problems to local treatment resources, including peer support/recovery groups. In addition, therapeutic work environments that provide employment for drug-abusing individuals who can demonstrate abstinence have been shown not only to promote a continued drug-free lifestyle but also to improve job skills, punctuality, and other behaviors necessary for active employment throughout life. Urine testing facilities, trained personnel, and workplace monitors are needed to implement this type of treatment.

What role can the criminal justice system play in addressing drug addiction?

It is estimated that about one-half of State and Federal prisoners abuse or are addicted to drugs, but relatively few receive treatment while incarcerated. Initiating drug abuse treatment in prison and continuing it upon release is vital to both individual recovery and to public health and safety. Various studies have shown that combining prison- and community-based treatment for addicted offenders reduces the risk of both recidivism to drug-related criminal behavior and relapse to drug use—which, in turn, nets huge savings in societal costs. A 2009 study in Baltimore, Maryland, for example, found that opioid-addicted prisoners who started methadone treatment (along with counseling) in prison and then continued it after release had better outcomes (reduced drug use and criminal activity) than those who only received counseling while in prison or those who only started methadone treatment after their release.

> Individuals who enter treatment under legal pressure have outcomes as favorable as those who enter treatment voluntarily.

The majority of offenders involved with the criminal justice system are not in prison but are under community supervision. For those with known drug problems, drug addiction treatment may be recommended or mandated as a condition of probation. Research has demonstrated that individuals who enter treatment under legal pressure have outcomes as favorable as those who enter treatment voluntarily.

The criminal justice system refers drug offenders into treatment through a variety of mechanisms, such as diverting nonviolent offenders to treatment; stipulating treatment as a condition of incarceration, probation, or pretrial release; and convening specialized courts, or drug courts, that handle drug offense cases. These courts mandate and arrange for treatment as an alternative to incarceration, actively monitor progress in treatment, and arrange for other services for drug-involved offenders.

The most effective models integrate criminal justice and drug treatment systems and services. Treatment and criminal justice personnel work together on treatment planning—including implementation of screening, placement, testing, monitoring, and supervision—as well as on the systematic use of sanctions and rewards. Treatment for incarcerated drug abusers should include continuing care, monitoring, and supervision after incarceration and during parole. Methods to achieve better coordination between parole/probation officers and health providers are being studied to improve offender outcomes. (For more information, please see NIDA's _Principles of Drug Abuse Treatment for Criminal Justice Populations: A Research-Based Guide_ [revised 2012].)

What are the unique needs of women with substance use disorders?

Gender-related drug abuse treatment should attend not only to biological differences but also to social and environmental factors, all of which can influence the motivations for drug use, the reasons for seeking treatment, the types of environments where treatment is obtained, the treatments that are most effective, and the consequences of not receiving treatment. Many life circumstances predominate in women as a group, which may require a specialized treatment approach. For example, research has shown that physical and sexual trauma followed by post-traumatic stress disorder (PTSD) is more common in drug-abusing women than in men seeking treatment. Other factors unique to women that can influence the treatment process include issues around how they come into treatment (as women are more likely than men to seek the assistance of a general or mental health practitioner), financial independence, and pregnancy and child care.

What are the unique needs of pregnant women with substance use disorders?

Using drugs, alcohol, or tobacco during pregnancy exposes not just the woman but also her developing fetus to the substance and can have potentially deleterious and even long-term effects on exposed children. Smoking during pregnancy can increase risk of stillbirth, infant mortality, sudden infant death syndrome, preterm birth, respiratory problems, slowed fetal growth, and low birth weight. Drinking during pregnancy can lead to the child developing fetal alcohol spectrum disorders, characterized by low birth weight and enduring cognitive and behavioral problems.

Prenatal use of some drugs, including opioids, may cause a withdrawal syndrome in newborns called neonatal abstinence syndrome (NAS). Babies with NAS are at greater risk of seizures, respiratory problems, feeding difficulties, low birth weight, and even death.

Research has established the value of evidence-based treatments for pregnant women (and their babies), including medications. For example, although no medications have been FDA-approved to treat opioid dependence in pregnant women, methadone maintenance combined with prenatal care and a comprehensive drug treatment program can improve many of the detrimental outcomes associated with untreated heroin abuse. However, newborns exposed to methadone during pregnancy still require treatment for withdrawal symptoms. Recently, another medication option for opioid dependence, buprenorphine, has been shown to produce fewer NAS symptoms in babies than methadone, resulting in shorter infant hospital stays. In general, it is important to closely monitor women who are trying to quit drug use during pregnancy and to provide treatment as needed.

What are the unique needs of adolescents with substance use disorders?

Adolescent drug abusers have unique needs stemming from their immature neurocognitive and psychosocial stage of development. Research has demonstrated that the brain undergoes a prolonged process of development and refinement from birth through early adulthood. Over the course of this developmental period, a young person's actions go from being more impulsive to being more reasoned and reflective. In fact, the brain areas most closely associated with aspects of behavior such as decision-making, judgment, planning, and self-control undergo a period of rapid development during adolescence and young adulthood.

Adolescent drug abuse is also often associated with other co-occurring mental health problems. These include attention-deficit hyperactivity disorder (ADHD), oppositional defiant disorder, and conduct problems, as well as depressive and anxiety disorders.

Adolescents are also especially sensitive to social cues, with peer groups and families being highly influential during this time. Therefore, treatments that facilitate positive parental involvement, integrate other systems in which the adolescent participates (such as school and athletics), and recognize the importance of prosocial peer relationships are among the most effective. Access to comprehensive assessment, treatment, case management, and family-support services that are developmentally, culturally, and gender-appropriate is also integral when addressing adolescent addiction.

Medications for substance abuse among adolescents may in certain cases be helpful. Currently, the only addiction medications approved by FDA for people under 18 are over-the-counter transdermal nicotine skin patches, chewing gum, and lozenges (physician advice should be sought first). Buprenorphine, a medication for treating opioid addiction that must be prescribed by specially trained physicians, has not been approved for adolescents, but recent research suggests it could be effective for those as young as 16. Studies are under way to determine the safety and efficacy of this and other medications for opioid-, nicotine-, and alcohol-dependent adolescents and for adolescents with co-occurring disorders.

Are there specific drug addiction treatments for older adults?

With the aging of the baby boomer generation, the composition of the general population is changing dramatically with respect to the number of older adults. Such a change, coupled with a greater history of lifetime drug use (than previous older generations), different cultural norms and general attitudes about drug use, and increases in the availability of psychotherapeutic medications, is already leading to greater drug use by older adults and may increase substance use problems in this population. While substance abuse in older adults often goes unrecognized and therefore untreated, research indicates that currently available addiction treatment programs can be as effective for them as for younger adults.

Can a person become addicted to medications prescribed by a doctor?

Yes. People who abuse prescription drugs—that is, taking them in a manner or a dose other than prescribed, or taking medications prescribed for another person—risk addiction and other serious health consequences. Such drugs include opioid pain relievers, stimulants used to treat ADHD, and benzodiazepines to treat anxiety or sleep disorders. Indeed, in 2010, an estimated 2.4 million people 12 or older met criteria for abuse of or dependence on prescription drugs, the second most common illicit drug use after marijuana. To minimize these risks, a physician (or other prescribing health provider) should screen patients for prior or current substance abuse problems and assess their family history of substance abuse or addiction before prescribing a psychoactive medication and monitor patients who are prescribed such drugs. Physicians also need to educate patients about the potential risks so that they will follow their physician's instructions faithfully, safeguard their medications, and dispose of them appropriately.

Is there a difference between physical dependence and addiction?

Yes. Addiction—or compulsive drug use despite harmful consequences—is characterized by an inability to stop using a drug; failure to meet work, social, or family obligations; and, sometimes (depending on the drug), tolerance and withdrawal. The latter reflect physical dependence in which the body adapts to the drug, requiring more of it to achieve a certain effect (tolerance) and eliciting drug-specific physical or mental symptoms if drug use is abruptly ceased (withdrawal). Physical dependence can happen with the chronic use of many drugs—including many prescription drugs, even if taken as instructed. Thus, physical dependence in and of itself does not constitute addiction, but it often accompanies addiction. This distinction can be difficult to discern, particularly with prescribed pain medications, for which the need for increasing dosages can represent tolerance or a worsening underlying problem, as opposed to the beginning of abuse or addiction.

How do other mental disorders coexisting with drug addiction affect drug addiction treatment?

Drug addiction is a disease of the brain that frequently occurs with other mental disorders. In fact, as many as 6 in 10 people with an illicit substance use disorder also suffer from another mental illness; and rates are similar for users of licit drugs—i.e., tobacco and alcohol. For these individuals, one condition becomes more difficult to treat successfully as an additional condition is intertwined. Thus, people entering treatment either for a substance use disorder or for another mental disorder should be assessed for the co-occurrence of the other condition. Research indicates that treating both (or multiple) illnesses simultaneously in an integrated fashion is generally the best treatment approach for these patients.

Is the use of medications like methadone and buprenorphine simply replacing one addiction with another?

No. Buprenorphine and methadone are prescribed or administered under monitored, controlled conditions and are safe and effective for treating opioid addiction when used as directed. They are administered orally or sublingually (i.e., under the tongue) in specified doses, and their effects differ from those of heroin and other abused opioids.

Heroin, for example, is often injected, snorted, or smoked, causing an almost immediate "rush," or brief period of intense euphoria, that wears off quickly and ends in a "crash." The individual then experiences an intense craving to use the drug again to stop the crash and reinstate the euphoria.

The cycle of euphoria, crash, and craving—sometimes repeated several times a day—is a hallmark of addiction and results in severe behavioral disruption. These characteristics result from heroin's rapid onset and short duration of action in the brain.

> As used in maintenance treatment, methadone and buprenorphine are not heroin/opioid substitutes.

In contrast, methadone and buprenorphine have gradual onsets of action and produce stable levels of the drug in the brain. As a result, patients maintained on these medications do not experience a rush, while they also markedly reduce their desire to use opioids.

If an individual treated with these medications tries to take an opioid such as heroin, the euphoric effects are usually dampened or suppressed. Patients undergoing maintenance treatment do not experience the physiological or behavioral abnormalities from rapid fluctuations in drug levels associated with heroin use. Maintenance treatments save lives—they help to stabilize individuals, allowing treatment of their medical, psychological, and other problems so they can contribute effectively as members of families and of society.

Where do 12-step or self-help programs fit into drug addiction treatment?

Self-help groups can complement and extend the effects of professional treatment. The most prominent self-help groups are those affiliated with Alcoholics Anonymous (AA), Narcotics Anonymous (NA), and Cocaine Anonymous (CA), all of which are based on the 12-step model. Most drug addiction treatment programs encourage patients to participate in self-help group therapy during and after formal treatment. These groups can be particularly helpful during recovery, offering an added layer of community-level social support to help people achieve and maintain abstinence and other healthy lifestyle behaviors over the course of a lifetime.

Can exercise play a role in the treatment process?

Yes. Exercise is increasingly becoming a component of many treatment programs and has proven effective, when combined with cognitive-behavioral therapy, at helping people quit smoking. Exercise may exert beneficial effects by addressing psychosocial and physiological needs that nicotine replacement alone does not, by reducing negative feelings and stress, and by helping prevent weight gain following cessation. Research to determine if and how exercise programs can play a similar role in the treatment of other forms of drug abuse is under way.

How does drug addiction treatment help reduce the spread of HIV/AIDS, Hepatitis C (HCV), and other infectious diseases?

Drug-abusing individuals, including injecting and non-injecting drug users, are at increased risk of human immunodeficiency virus (HIV), hepatitis C virus (HCV), and other infectious diseases. These diseases are transmitted by sharing contaminated drug injection equipment and by engaging in risky sexual behavior sometimes associated with drug use. Effective drug abuse treatment is HIV/HCV prevention because it reduces activities that can spread disease, such as sharing injection equipment and engaging in unprotected sexual activity. Counseling that targets a range of HIV/HCV risk behaviors provides an added level of disease prevention.

> Drug abuse treatment is HIV and HCV prevention.

Injection drug users who do not enter treatment are up to six times more likely to become infected with HIV than those who enter and remain in treatment. Participation in treatment also presents opportunities for HIV screening and referral to early HIV treatment. In fact, recent research from NIDA's National Drug Abuse Treatment Clinical Trials Network showed that providing rapid onsite HIV testing in substance abuse treatment facilities increased patients' likelihood of being tested and of receiving their test results. HIV counseling and testing are key aspects of superior drug abuse treatment programs and should be offered to all individuals entering treatment. Greater availability of inexpensive and unobtrusive rapid HIV tests should increase access to these important aspects of HIV prevention and treatment.

Drug Addiction Treatment in the United States

> Treatment for drug abuse and addiction is delivered in many different settings, using a variety of behavioral and pharmacological approaches.

Drug addiction is a complex disorder that can involve virtually every aspect of an individual's functioning—in the family, at work and school, and in the community.

Because of addiction's complexity and pervasive consequences, drug addiction treatment typically must involve many components. Some of those components focus directly on the individual's drug use; others, like employment training, focus on restoring the addicted individual to productive membership in the family and society (See diagram "Components of Comprehensive Drug Abuse Treatment"), enabling him or her to experience the rewards associated with abstinence.

Treatment for drug abuse and addiction is delivered in many different settings using a variety of behavioral and pharmacological approaches. In the United States, more than 14,500 specialized drug treatment facilities provide counseling, behavioral therapy, medication, case management, and other types of services to persons with substance use disorders.

Along with specialized drug treatment facilities, drug abuse and addiction are treated in physicians' offices and mental health clinics by a variety of providers, including counselors, physicians, psychiatrists, psychologists, nurses, and social workers. Treatment is delivered in outpatient, inpatient, and residential settings. Although specific treatment approaches often are associated with particular treatment settings, a variety of therapeutic interventions or services can be included in any given setting.

Because drug abuse and addiction are major public health problems, a large portion of drug treatment is funded by local, State, and Federal governments. Private and employer-subsidized health plans also may provide coverage for treatment of addiction and its medical consequences. Unfortunately, managed care has resulted in shorter average stays, while a historical lack of or insufficient coverage for substance abuse treatment has curtailed the number of operational programs. The recent passage of parity for insurance coverage of mental health and substance abuse problems will hopefully improve this state of affairs. Health Care Reform (i.e., the Patient Protection and Affordable Care Act of 2010, "ACA") also stands to increase the demand for drug abuse treatment services and presents an opportunity to study how innovations in service delivery, organization, and financing can improve access to and use of them.

Types of Treatment Programs

Research studies on addiction treatment typically have classified programs into several general types or modalities. Treatment approaches and individual programs continue to evolve and diversify, and many programs today do not fit neatly into traditional drug adiction treatment classifications.

Most, however, start with detoxification and medically managed withdrawal, often considered the first stage of treatment. Detoxification, the process by which the body clears itself of drugs, is designed to manage the acute and potentially dangerous physiological effects of stopping drug use. As stated previously, detoxification alone does not address the psychological, social, and behavioral problems associated with addiction and therefore does not typically produce lasting behavioral changes necessary for recovery. Detoxification should thus be followed by a formal assessment and referral to drug addiction treatment.

Because it is often accompanied by unpleasant and potentially fatal side effects stemming from withdrawal, detoxification is often managed with medications administered by a physician in an inpatient or outpatient setting; therefore, it is referred to as "medically managed withdrawal." Medications are available to assist in the withdrawal from opioids, benzodiazepines, alcohol, nicotine, barbiturates, and other sedatives.

Further Reading:

Kleber, H.D. Outpatient detoxification from opiates. *Primary Psychiatry* 1:42-52, 1996.

Long-Term Residential Treatment

Long-term residential treatment provides care 24 hours a day, generally in non-hospital settings. The best-known residential treatment model is the therapeutic community (TC), with planned lengths of stay of between 6 and 12 months. TCs focus on the "resocialization" of the individual and use the program's entire community—including other residents, staff, and the social context—as active components of treatment. Addiction is viewed in the context of an individual's social and psychological deficits, and treatment focuses on developing personal accountability and responsibility as well as socially productive lives. Treatment is highly structured and can be confrontational at times, with activities designed to help residents examine damaging beliefs, self-concepts, and destructive patterns of behavior and adopt new, more harmonious and constructive ways to interact with others. Many TCs offer comprehensive services, which can include employment training and other support services, onsite. Research shows that TCs can be modified to treat individuals with special needs, including adolescents, women, homeless individuals, people with severe mental disorders, and individuals in the criminal justice system (see "Treating Criminal Justice-Involved Drug Abusers and Addicted Individuals").

Further Reading:

Lewis, B.F.; McCusker, J.; Hindin, R.; Frost, R.; and Garfield, F. Four residential drug treatment programs: Project IMPACT. In: J.A. Inciardi, F.M. Tims, and B.W. Fletcher (eds.), *Innovative Approaches in the Treatment of Drug Abuse*, Westport, CT: Greenwood Press, pp. 45-60, 1993.

Sacks, S.; Banks, S.; McKendrick, K.; and Sacks, J.Y. Modified therapeutic community for co-occurring disorders: A summary of four studies. *Journal of*

Substance Abuse Treatment 34(1):112-122, 2008.

Sacks, S.; Sacks, J.; DeLeon, G.; Bernhardt, A.; and Staines, G. Modified therapeutic community for mentally ill chemical "abusers": Background; influences; program description; preliminary findings. *Substance Use and Misuse* 32(9):1217-1259, 1997.

Stevens, S.J., and Glider, P.J. Therapeutic communities: Substance abuse treatment for women. In: F.M. Tims, G. DeLeon, and N. Jainchill (eds.), *Therapeutic Community: Advances in Research and Application,* National Institute on Drug Abuse Research Monograph 144, NIH Pub. No. 94-3633, U.S. Government Printing Office, pp. 162-180, 1994.

Sullivan, C.J.; McKendrick, K.; Sacks, S.; and Banks, S.M. Modified therapeutic community for offenders with MICA disorders: Substance use outcomes. *American Journal of Drug and Alcohol Abuse* 33(6):823-832, 2007.

Short-Term Residential Treatment

Short-term residential programs provide intensive but relatively brief treatment based on a modified 12-step approach. These programs were originally designed to treat alcohol problems, but during the cocaine epidemic of the mid-1980s, many began to treat other types of substance use disorders. The original residential treatment model consisted of a 3- to 6-week hospital-based inpatient treatment phase followed by extended outpatient therapy and participation in a self-help group, such as AA. Following stays in residential treatment programs, it is important for individuals to remain engaged in outpatient treatment programs and/or aftercare programs. These programs help to reduce the risk of relapse once a patient leaves the residential setting.

Further Reading:

Hubbard, R.L.; Craddock, S.G.; Flynn, P.M.; Anderson, J.; and Etheridge, R.M. Overview of 1-year follow-up outcomes in the Drug Abuse Treatment Outcome Study (DATOS). *Psychology of Addictive Behaviors* 11(4):291-298, 1998.

Miller, M.M. Traditional approaches to the treatment of addiction. In: A.W. Graham and T.K. Schultz (eds.), *Principles of Addiction Medicine* (2nd ed.). Washington, D.C.: American Society of Addiction Medicine, 1998.

Outpatient Treatment Programs

Outpatient treatment varies in the types and intensity of services offered. Such treatment costs less than residential or inpatient treatment and often is more suitable for people with jobs or extensive social supports. It should be noted, however, that low-intensity programs may offer little more than drug education. Other outpatient models, such as intensive day treatment, can be comparable to residential programs in services and effectiveness, depending on the individual patient's characteristics and needs. In many outpatient programs, group counseling can be a major component. Some outpatient programs are also designed to treat patients with medical or other mental health problems in addition to their drug disorders.

Further Reading:

Hubbard, R.L.; Craddock, S.G.; Flynn, P.M.; Anderson, J.; and Etheridge, R.M. Overview of 1-year follow-up outcomes in the Drug Abuse Treatment Outcome Study (DATOS). *Psychology of Addictive Behaviors* 11(4):291-298, 1998.

Institute of Medicine. *Treating Drug Problems.* Washington, D.C.: National Academy Press, 1990.

McLellan, A.T.; Grisson, G.; Durell, J.; Alterman, A.I.; Brill, P.; and O'Brien, C.P. Substance abuse treatment in the private setting: Are some programs more effective than others? *Journal of Substance Abuse Treatment* 10:243-254, 1993.

Simpson, D.D., and Brown, B.S. Treatment retention and follow-up outcomes in the Drug Abuse Treatment Outcome Study (DATOS). *Psychology of Addictive Behaviors* 11(4):294-307, 1998.

Individualized Drug Counseling

Individualized drug counseling not only focuses on reducing or stopping illicit drug or alcohol use; it also addresses related areas of impaired functioning—such as employment status, illegal activity, and family/social relations—as well as the content and structure of the patient's recovery program. Through its emphasis on short-term behavioral goals, individualized counseling helps the patient develop coping strategies and tools to abstain from drug use and maintain abstinence. The addiction counselor encourages 12-step participation (at least one or two times per week) and makes referrals for needed supplemental medical, psychiatric, employment, and other services.

Group Counseling

Many therapeutic settings use group therapy to capitalize on the social reinforcement offered by peer discussion and to help promote drug-free lifestyles. Research has shown that when group therapy either is offered in conjunction with individualized drug counseling or is formatted to reflect the principles of cognitive-behavioral therapy or contingency management, positive outcomes are achieved. Currently, researchers are testing conditions in which group therapy can be standardized and made more community-friendly.

Treating Criminal Justice-Involved Drug Abusers and Addicted Individuals

Often, drug abusers come into contact with the criminal justice system earlier than other health or social systems, presenting opportunities for intervention and treatment prior to, during, after, or in lieu of incarceration. Research has shown that combining criminal justice sanctions with drug treatment can be effective in decreasing drug abuse and related crime. Individuals under legal coercion tend to stay in treatment longer and do as well as or better than those not under legal pressure. Studies show that for incarcerated individuals with drug problems, starting drug abuse treatment in prison and continuing the same treatment upon release—in other words, a seamless continuum of services—results in better outcomes: less drug use and less criminal behavior. More information on how the criminal justice system can address the problem of drug addiction can be found in Principles of Drug Abuse Treatment for Criminal Justice Populations: A Research-Based Guide (National Institute on Drug Abuse, revised 2012).

Treating Criminal Justice-Involved Drug Abusers and Addicted Individuals

Often, drug abusers come into contact with the criminal justice system earlier than other health or social systems, presenting opportunities for intervention and treatment prior to, during, after, or in lieu of incarceration. Research has shown that combining criminal justice sanctions with drug treatment can be effective in decreasing drug abuse and related crime. Individuals under legal coercion tend to stay in treatment longer and do as well as or better than those not under legal pressure. Studies show that for incarcerated individuals with drug problems, starting drug abuse treatment in prison and continuing the same treatment upon release—in other words, a seamless continuum of services—results in better outcomes: less drug use and less criminal behavior. More information on how the criminal justice system can address the problem of drug addiction can be found in Principles of Drug Abuse Treatment for Criminal Justice Populations: A Research-Based Guide (National Institute on Drug Abuse, revised 2012).

Evidence-Based Approaches to Drug Addiction Treatment

> Each approach to drug treatment is designed to address certain aspects of drug addiction and its consequences for the individual, family, and society.

This section presents examples of treatment approaches and components that have an evidence base supporting their use. Each approach is designed to address certain aspects of drug addiction and its consequences for the individual, family, and society. Some of the approaches are intended to supplement or enhance existing treatment programs, and others are fairly comprehensive in and of themselves.

The following section is broken down into Pharmacotherapies, Behavioral Therapies, and Behavioral Therapies Primarily for Adolescents. They are further subdivided according to particular substance use disorders. This list is not exhaustive, and new treatments are continually under development.

Pharmacotherapies

Opioid Addiction

Methadone

Methadone is a long-acting synthetic opioid agonist medication that can prevent withdrawal symptoms and reduce craving in opioid-addicted individuals. It can also block the effects of illicit opioids. It has a long history of use in treatment of opioid dependence in adults and is taken orally. Methadone maintenance treatment is available in all but three States through specially licensed opioid treatment programs or methadone maintenance programs.

Combined with behavioral treatment: Research has shown that methadone maintenance is more effective when it includes individual and/or group counseling, with even better outcomes when patients are provided with, or referred to, other needed medical/psychiatric, psychological, and social services (e.g., employment or family services).

Further Reading:

Dole, V.P.; Nyswander, M.; and Kreek, M.J. Narcotic blockade. *Archives of Internal Medicine* 118:304–309, 1966.

McLellan, A.T.; Arndt, I.O.; Metzger, D.; Woody, G.E.; and O'Brien, C.P. The effects of psychosocial services in substance abuse treatment. *The Journal of the American Medical Association* 269(15):1953–1959, 1993.

The Rockerfeller University. The first pharmacological treatment for narcotic addiction: Methadone maintenance. The Rockefeller University Hospital Centennial, 2010. Available at centennial.rucares.org/index.php?page=Methadone_Maintenance.

Woody, G.E.; Luborsky, L.; McClellan, A.T.; O'Brien, C.P.; Beck, A.T.; Blaine, J.; Herman, I.; and Hole, A. Psychotherapy for opiate addicts: Does it help? *Archives of General Psychiatry* 40:639–645, 1983.

Buprenorphine

Buprenorphine is a synthetic opioid medication that acts as a partial agonist at opioid receptors—it does not produce the euphoria and sedation caused by heroin or other opioids but is able to reduce or eliminate withdrawal symptoms associated with opioid dependence and carries a low risk of overdose.

Buprenorphine is currently available in two formulations that are taken sublingually: (1) a pure form of the drug and (2) a more commonly prescribed formulation called Suboxone, which combines buprenorphine with the drug naloxone, an antagonist (or blocker) at opioid receptors. Naloxone has no effect when Suboxone is taken as prescribed, but if an addicted individual attempts to inject Suboxone, the naloxone will produce severe withdrawal symptoms. Thus, this formulation lessens the likelihood that the drug will be abused or diverted to others.

Buprenorphine treatment for detoxification and/or maintenance can be provided in office-based settings by qualified physicians who have received a waiver from the Drug Enforcement Administration (DEA), allowing them to prescribe it. The availability of office-based treatment for opioid addiction is a cost-effective approach that increases the reach of treatment and the options available to patients.

Buprenorphine is also available as in an implant and injection. The U.S. Food and Drug Administration (FDA) approved a 6-month subdermal buprenorphine implant in May 2016 and a once-monthly buprenorphine injection in November 2017.

Further Reading:

Fiellin, D.A.; Pantalon, M.V.; Chawarski, M.C.; Moore, B.A.; Sullivan, L.E.; O'Connor, P.G.; and Schottenfeld, R.S. Counseling plus buprenorphine/naloxone maintenance therapy for opioid dependence. *The New England Journal of Medicine* 355(4):365–374, 2006.

Fudala P.J.; Bridge, T.P.; Herbert, S.; Williford, W.O.; Chiang, C.N.; Jones, K.; Collins, J.; Raisch, D.; Casadonte, P.; Goldsmith, R.J.; Ling, W.; Malkerneker, U.; McNicholas, L.; Renner, J.; Stine, S.; and Tusel, D. for the Buprenorphine/Naloxone Collaborative Study Group. Office-based treatment of opiate addiction with a sublingual-tablet formulation of buprenorphine and naloxone. *The New England Journal of Medicine* 349(10):949–958, 2003.

Kosten, T.R.; and Fiellin, D.A. U.S. National Buprenorphine Implementation Program: Buprenorphine for office-based practice. Consensus conference overview. *The American Journal on Addictions* 13(Suppl. 1):S1–S7, 2004.

McCance-Katz, E.F. Office-based buprenorphine treatment for opioid-dependent patients. *Harvard Review of Psychiatry* 12(6):321–338, 2004.

> **Treatment, not Substitution**
>
> Because methadone and buprenorphine are themselves opioids, some people view these treatments for opioid dependence as just substitutions of one addictive drug for another (see Question 19). But taking these medications as prescribed allows patients to hold jobs, avoid street crime and violence, and reduce their exposure to HIV by stopping or decreasing injection drug use and drug-related high-risk sexual behavior. Patients stabilized on these medications can also engage more readily in counseling and other behavioral interventions essential to recovery.

Naltrexone

Naltrexone is a synthetic opioid antagonist—it blocks opioids from binding to their receptors and thereby prevents their euphoric and other effects. It has been used for many years to reverse opioid overdose and is also approved for treating opioid addiction. The theory behind this treatment is that the repeated absence of the desired effects and the perceived futility of abusing opioids will gradually diminish craving and addiction. Naltrexone itself has no subjective effects following detoxification (that is, a person does not perceive any particular drug effect), it has no potential for abuse, and it is not addictive.

Naltrexone as a treatment for opioid addiction is usually prescribed in outpatient medical settings, although the treatment should begin after medical detoxification in a residential setting in order to prevent withdrawal symptoms.

Naltrexone must be taken orally—either daily or three times a week—but noncompliance with treatment is a common problem. Many experienced clinicians have found naltrexone best suited for highly motivated, recently detoxified patients who desire total abstinence because of external circumstances—for instance, professionals or parolees. Recently, a long-acting injectable version of naltrexone, called Vivitrol, was approved to treat opioid addiction. Because it only needs to be delivered once a month, this version of the drug can facilitate compliance and offers an alternative for those who do not wish to be placed on agonist/partial agonist medications.

Further Reading:

Cornish, J.W.; Metzger, D.; Woody, G.E.; Wilson, D.; McClellan, A.T.; and Vandergrift, B. Naltrexone pharmacotherapy for opioid dependent federal probationers. *Journal of Substance Abuse Treatment* 14(6):529–534, 1997.

Gastfriend, D.R. Intramuscular extended-release naltrexone: current evidence. *Annals of the New York Academy of Sciences* 1216:144–166, 2011.

Krupitsky, E.; Illerperuma, A.; Gastfriend, D.R.; and Silverman, B.L. Efficacy and safety of extended-release injectable naltrexone (XR-NTX) for the treatment of opioid dependence. Paper presented at the 2010 annual meeting of the American Psychiatric Association, New Orleans, LA.

Comparing Buprenorphine and Naltrexone

A NIDA study comparing the effectiveness of a buprenorphine/naloxone combination and an extended release naltrexone formulation on treating opioid use disorder has found that both medications are similarly effective in treating opioid use disorder once treatment is initiated. Because naltrexone requires full detoxification, initiating treatment among active opioid users was more difficult with this medication. However, once detoxification was complete, the naltrexone formulation had a similar effectiveness as the buprenorphine/naloxone combination.

Tobacco Addiction

Nicotine Replacement Therapy (NRT)

A variety of formulations of nicotine replacement therapies (NRTs) now exist, including the transdermal nicotine patch, nicotine spray, nicotine gum, and nicotine lozenges. Because nicotine is the main addictive ingredient in tobacco, the rationale for NRT is that stable low levels of nicotine will prevent withdrawal symptoms—which often drive continued tobacco use—and help keep people motivated to quit. Research shows that combining the patch with another replacement therapy is more effective than a single therapy alone.

Bupropion (Zyban®)

Bupropion was originally marketed as an antidepressant (Wellbutrin). It produces mild stimulant effects by blocking the reuptake of certain neurotransmitters, especially norepinephrine and dopamine. A serendipitous observation among depressed patients was that the medication was also effective in suppressing tobacco craving, helping them quit smoking without also gaining weight. Although bupropion's exact mechanisms of action in facilitating smoking cessation are unclear, it has FDA approval as a smoking cessation treatment.

Varenicline (Chantix®)

Varenicline is the most recently FDA-approved medication for smoking cessation. It acts on a subset of nicotinic receptors in the brain thought to be involved in the rewarding effects of nicotine. Varenicline acts as a partial agonist/antagonist at these receptors—this means that it midly stimulates the nicotine receptor but not sufficiently to trigger the release of dopamine, which is important for the rewarding effects of nicotine. As an antagonist, varenicline also blocks the ability of nicotine to activate dopamine, interfering with the reinforcing effects of smoking, thereby reducing cravings and supporting abstinence from smoking.

Combined With Behavioral Treatment

Each of the above pharmacotherapies is recommended for use in combination with behavioral interventions, including group and individual therapies, as well as telephone quitlines. Behavioral approaches complement most tobacco addiction treatment programs. They can amplify the effects of medications by teaching people how to manage stress, recognize and avoid high-risk situations for smoking relapse, and develop alternative coping strategies (e.g., cigarette refusal skills, assertiveness, and time management skills) that they can practice in treatment, social, and work settings. Combined treatment is urged because behavioral and pharmacological treatments are thought to operate by different yet complementary mechanisms that can have additive effects.

Further Reading:

Alterman, A.I.; Gariti, P.; and Mulvaney, F. Short- and long-term smoking cessation for three levels of intensity of behavioral treatment. *Psychology of Addictive Behaviors* 15:261-264, 2001.

Hall, S.M.; Humfleet, G.L.; Muñoz, R.F.; V.I; Prochaska, J.J.; and Robbins, J.A. Using extended cognitive behavioral treatment and medication to treat dependent smokers. *American Journal of Public Health* 101:2349–2356, 2011.

Jorenby, D.E.; Hays, J.T.; Rigotti, N.A.; Azoulay, S.; Watsky, E.J.; Williams, K.E.; Billing, C.B.; Gong, J.; and Reeves, K.R. Varenicline Phase 3 Study Group. Efficacy of varenicline, an 42 nicotinic acetylcholine receptor partial agonist vs. placebo or sustained-release bupropion for smoking cessation: A randomized controlled trial. *The Journal of the American Medical Association* 296(1):56–63, 2006.

King, D.P.; Paciqa, S.; Pickering, E.; Benowitz, N.L.; Bierut, L.J.; Conti, D.V.; Kaprio, J.; Lerman, C.; and Park, P.W. Smoking cessation pharmacogenetics: Analysis of varenicline and bupropion in placebo-controlled clinical trials. *Neuropsychopharmacology* 37:641–650, 2012.

Raupach, T.; and van Schayck, C.P. Pharmacotherapy for smoking cessation: Current advances and research topics. *CNS Drugs* 25:371–382, 2011.

Shah, S.D.; Wilken, L.A.; Winkler, S.R.; and Lin, S.J. Systematic review and meta-analysis of combination therapy for smoking cessation. *Journal of the American Pharmaceutical Association* 48(5):659–665, 2008.

Smith, S.S; McCarthy, D.E.; Japuntich S.J.; Christiansen, B.; Piper, M.E.; Jorenby, D.E.; Fraser, D.L.; Fiore, M.C.; Baker, T.B.; and Jackson, T.C. Comparative effectiveness of 5 smoking cessation pharmacotherapies in primary care clinics. *Archives of Internal Medicine* 169:2148–2155, 2009.

Stitzer, M. Combined behavioral and pharmacological treatments for smoking cessation. *Nicotine & Tobacco Research* 1:S181–S187, 1999.

Alcohol Addiction

Naltrexone

Naltrexone blocks opioid receptors that are involved in the rewarding effects of drinking and the craving for alcohol. It has been shown to reduce relapse to problem drinking in some patients. An extended release version, Vivitrol—administered once a month by injection—is also FDA-approved for treating alcoholism, and may offer benefits regarding compliance.

Acamprosate

Acamprosate (Campral®) acts on the gamma-aminobutyric acid (GABA) and glutamate neurotransmitter systems and is thought to reduce symptoms of protracted withdrawal, such as insomnia, anxiety, restlessness, and dysphoria. Acamprosate has been shown to help dependent drinkers maintain abstinence for several weeks to months, and it may be more effective in patients with severe dependence.

Disulfiram

Disulfiram (Antabuse®) interferes with degradation of alcohol, resulting in the accumulation of acetaldehyde, which, in turn, produces a very unpleasant reaction that includes flushing, nausea, and plapitations if a person drinks alcohol. The utility and effectiveness of disulfiram are considered limited because compliance is generally poor. However, among patients who are highly motivated, disulfiram can be effective, and some patients use it episodically for high-risk situations, such as social occasions where alcohol is present. It can also be administered in a monitored fashion, such as in a clinic or by a spouse, improving its efficacy.

Topiramate

Topiramate is thought to work by increasing inhibitory (GABA) neurotransmission and reducing stimulatory (glutamate) neurotransmission, although its precise mechanism of action is not known. Although topiramate has not yet received FDA approval for treating alcohol addiction, it is sometimes used off-label for this purpose. Topiramate has been shown in studies to significantly improve multiple drinking outcomes, compared with a placebo.

Combined With Behavioral Treatment

While a number of behavioral treatments have been shown to be effective in the treatment of alcohol addiction, it does not appear that an additive effect exists between behavioral treatments and pharmacotherapy. Studies have shown that just getting help is one of the most important factors in treating alcohol addiction; the precise type of treatment received is not as important.

Further Reading:

Anton, R.F.; O'Malley, S.S.; Ciraulo, D.A.; Cisler, R.A.; Couper, D.; Donovan, D.M.; Gastfriend, D.R.; Hosking, J.D.; Johnson, B.A.; LoCastro, J.S.; Longabaugh, R.; Mason, B.J.; Mattson, M.E.; Miller, W.R.; Pettinati, H.M.; Randall, C.L.; Swift, R.; Weiss, R.D.; Williams, L.D.; and Zweben, A., for the COMBINE Study Research Group. Combined pharmacotherapies and behavioral interventions for alcohol dependence: The COMBINE study: A randomized controlled trial. *The Journal of the American Medical Association* 295(17):2003–2017, 2006.

National Institute on Alcohol Abuse and Alcoholism. Helping Patients Who Drink Too Much: A Clinician's Guide, Updated 2005 Edition. Bethesda, MD: NIAAA, updated 2005. Available at
pubs.niaaa.nih.gov/publications/Practitioner/CliniciansGuide2005/clinicians_guide.htm

Behavioral Therapies

Behavioral approaches help engage people in drug abuse treatment, provide incentives for them to remain abstinent, modify their attitudes and behaviors related to drug abuse, and increase their life skills to handle stressful circumstances and environmental cues that may trigger intense craving for drugs and prompt another cycle of compulsive abuse. Below are a number of behavioral therapies shown to be effective in addressing substance abuse (effectiveness with particular drugs of abuse is denoted in parentheses).

Cognitive-Behavioral Therapy (Alcohol, Marijuana, Cocaine, Methamphetamine, Nicotine)

Cognitive-Behavioral Therapy (CBT) was developed as a method to prevent relapse when treating problem drinking, and later it was adapted for cocaine-addicted individuals. Cognitive-behavioral strategies are based on the theory that in the development of maladaptive behavioral patterns like substance abuse, learning processes play a critical role. Individuals in CBT learn to identify and correct problematic behaviors by applying a range of different skills that can be used to stop drug abuse and to address a range of other problems that often co-occur with it.

A central element of CBT is anticipating likely problems and enhancing patients' self-control by helping them develop effective coping strategies. Specific techniques include exploring the positive and negative consequences of continued drug use, self-monitoring to recognize cravings early and identify situations that might put one at risk for use, and developing strategies for coping with cravings and avoiding those high-risk situations.

Research indicates that the skills individuals learn through cognitive-behavioral approaches remain after the completion of treatment. Current research focuses on how to produce even more powerful effects by combining CBT with medications for drug abuse and with other types of behavioral therapies. A computer-based CBT system has also been developed and has been shown to be effective in helping reduce drug use following standard drug abuse treatment.

Further Reading:

Carroll, K.M., Easton, C.J.; Nich, C.; Hunkele, K.A.; Neavins, T.M.; Sinha, R.; Ford, H.L.; Vitolo, S.A; Doebrick, C.A.; and Rounsaville, B.J. The use of contingency management and motivational/skills-building therapy to treat young adults with marijuana dependence. *Journal of Consulting and Clinical Psychology* 74(5):955–966, 2006.

Carroll, K.M.; and Onken, L.S. Behavioral therapies for drug abuse. *The American Journal of Psychiatry* 168(8):1452–1460, 2005.

Carroll, K.M.; Sholomskas, D.; Syracuse, G.; Ball, S.A.; Nuro, K.; and Fenton, L.R. We don't train in vain: A dissemination trial of three strategies of training clinicians in cognitive-behavioral therapy. *Journal of Consulting and Clinical Psychology* 73(1):106–115, 2005.

Carroll, K.; Fenton, L.R.; Ball, S.A.; Nich, C.; Frankforter, T.L.; Shi,J.; and Rounsaville, B.J. Efficacy of disulfiram and cognitive behavior therapy in cocaine-dependent outpatients: A randomized placebo-controlled trial. *Archives of General Psychiatry* 61(3):264–272, 2004.

Carroll, K.M.; Ball, S.A.; Martino, S.; Nich, C.; Babuscio, T.A.; Nuro, K.F.; Gordon, M.A.; Portnoy, G.A.; and Rounsaville, B.J. Computer-assisted delivery of cognitive-behavioral therapy for addiction: a randomized trial of CBT4CBT. *The American Journal of Psychiatry* 165(7):881–888, 2008.

Contingency Management Interventions/Motivational Incentives (Alcohol, Stimulants, Opioids, Marijuana, Nicotine)

Research has demonstrated the effectiveness of treatment approaches using contingency management (CM) principles, which involve giving patients tangible rewards to reinforce positive behaviors such as abstinence. Studies conducted in both methadone programs and psychosocial counseling treatment programs demonstrate that incentive-based interventions are highly effective in increasing treatment retention and promoting abstinence from drugs.

Voucher-Based Reinforcement (VBR) augments other community-based treatments for adults who primarily abuse opioids (especially heroin) or stimulants (especially cocaine) or both. In VBR, the patient receives a voucher for every drug-free urine sample provided. The voucher has monetary value that can be exchanged for food items, movie passes, or other goods or services that are consistent with a drug-free lifestyle. The voucher values are low at first, but increase as the number of consecutive drug-free urine samples increases; positive urine samples reset the value of the vouchers to the initial low value. VBR has been shown to be effective in promoting abstinence from opioids and cocaine in patients undergoing methadone detoxification.

Prize Incentives CM applies similar principles as VBR but uses chances to win cash prizes instead of vouchers. Over the course of the program (at least 3 months, one or more times weekly), participants supplying drug-negative urine or breath tests draw from a bowl for the chance to win a prize worth between $1 and $100. Participants may also receive draws for attending counseling sessions and completing weekly goal-related activities. The number of draws starts at one and increases with consecutive negative drug tests and/or counseling sessions attended but resets to one with any drug-positive sample or unexcused absence. The practitioner community has raised concerns that this intervention could promote gambling—as it contains an element of chance—and that pathological gambling and substance use disorders can be comorbid. However, studies examining this concern found that Prize Incentives CM did not promote gambling behavior.

Further Reading:

Budney, A.J.; Moore, B.A.; Rocha, H.L.; and Higgins, S.T. Clinical trial of abstinence-based vouchers and cognitivebehavioral therapy for cannabis dependence. *Journal of Consulting and Clinical Psychology* 74(2):307–316, 2006.

Budney, A.J.; Roffman, R.; Stephens, R.S.; and Walker, D. Marijuana dependence and its treatment. *Addiction Science & Clinical Practice* 4(1):4–16, 2007.

Elkashef, A.; Vocci, F.; Huestis, M.; Haney, M.; Budney, A.; Gruber, A.; and el-Guebaly, N. Marijuana neurobiology and treatment. *Substance Abuse* 29(3):17–29, 2008.

Peirce, J.M.; Petry, N.M.; Stitzer, M.L.; Blaine, J.; Kellogg, S.; Satterfield, F.; Schwartz, M.; Krasnansky, J.; Pencer, E.; Silva-Vazquez, L.; Kirby, K.C.; Royer-Malvestuto, C.; Cohen, A.; Copersino, M.L.; Kolodner, K.; and Li, R. Effects of lower-cost incentives on stimulant abstinence in methadone maintenance treatment: A National Drug Abuse Treatment Clinical Trials Network study. *Archives of General Psychiatry* 63(2):201–208, 2006.

Petry, N.M.; Peirce, J.M.; Stitzer, M.L.; Blaine, J.; Roll, J.M.; Cohen, A.; Obert, J.; Killeen, T.; Saladin, M.E.; Cowell, M.; Kirby, K.C.; Sterling, R.; Royer-Malvestuto, C.; Hamilton, J.; Booth, R.E.; Macdonald, M.; Liebert, M.; Rader, L.; Burns, R; DiMaria, J.; Copersino, M.; Stabile, P.Q.; Kolodner, K.; and Li, R. Effect of prizebased incentives on outcomes in stimulant abusers in outpatient psychosocial treatment programs: A National Drug Abuse Treatment Clinical Trials Network study. *Archives of General Psychiatry* 62(10):1148–1156, 2005.

Petry, N.M.; Kolodner, K.B.; Li, R.; Peirce, J.M.; Roll, J.M.; Stitzer, M.L.; and Hamilton, J.A. Prize-based contingency management does not increase gambling. *Drug and Alcohol Dependence* 83(3):269–273, 2006.

Prendergast, M.; Podus, D.; Finney, J.; Greenwell, L.; and Roll, J. Contingency management for treatment of substance use disorders: A meta-analysis. *Addiction* 101(11):1546–1560, 2006.

Roll, J.M.; Petry, N.M.; Stitzer, M.L.; Brecht, M.L.; Peirce, J.M.; McCann, M.J.; Blaine, J.; MacDonald, M.; DiMaria, J.; Lucero, L.; and Kellogg, S. Contingency management for the treatment of methamphetamine use disorders. *The American Journal of Psychiatry* 163(11):1993–1999, 2006.

Community Reinforcement Approach Plus Vouchers (Alcohol, Cocaine, Opioids)

Community Reinforcement Approach (CRA) Plus Vouchers is an intensive 24-week outpatient therapy for treating people addicted to cocaine and alcohol. It uses a range of recreational, familial, social, and vocational reinforcers, along with material incentives, to make a non-drug-using lifestyle more rewarding than substance use. The treatment goals are twofold:

- To maintain abstinence long enough for patients to learn new life skills to help sustain it; and

- To reduce alcohol consumption for patients whose drinking is associated with cocaine use

Patients attend one or two individual counseling sessions each week, where they focus on improving family relations, learn a variety of skills to minimize drug use, receive vocational counseling, and develop new recreational activities and social networks. Those who also abuse alcohol receive clinic-monitored disulfiram (Antabuse) therapy. Patients submit urine samples two or three times each week and receive vouchers for cocaine-negative samples. As in VBR, the value of the vouchers increases with consecutive clean samples, and the vouchers may be exchanged for retail goods that are consistent with a drug-free lifestyle. Studies in both urban and rural areas have found that this approach facilitates patients' engagement in treatment and successfully aids them in gaining substantial periods of cocaine abstinence.

A computer-based version of CRA Plus Vouchers called the Therapeutic Education System (TES) was found to be nearly as effective as treatment administered by a therapist in promoting abstinence from opioids and cocaine among opioid-dependent individuals in outpatient treatment. A version of CRA for adolescents addresses problem-solving, coping, and communication skills and encourages active participation in positive social and recreational activities.

Further Reading:

Brooks, A.C.; Ryder, D.; Carise, D.; and Kirby, K.C. Feasibility and effectiveness of computer-based therapy in community treatment. *Journal of Substance Abuse Treatment* 39(3):227–235, 2010.

Higgins, S.T.; Sigmon, S.C.; Wong, C.J.; Heil, S.H.; Badger, G.J.; Donham, R.; Dantona, R.L.; and Anthony, S. Community reinforcement therapy for cocaine-dependent outpatients. *Archives of General Psychiatry* 60(10):1043–1052, 2003.

Roozen, H.G.; Boulogne, J.J.; van Tulder, M.W.; van den Brink, W.; De Jong, C.A.J.; and Kerhof, J.F.M. A systemic review of the effectiveness of the community reinforcement approach in alcohol, cocaine and opioid addiction. *Drug and Alcohol Dependence* 74(1):1–13, 2004.

Silverman, K.; Higgins, S.T.; Brooner, R.K.; Montoya, I.D.; Cone, E.J.; Schuster, C.R.; and Preston, K.L. Sustained cocaine abstinence in methadone maintenance patients through voucher-based reinforcement therapy. *Archives of General Psychiatry* 53(5):409–415, 1996.

Smith, J.E.; Meyers, R.J.; and Delaney, H.D. The community reinforcement approach with homeless alcohol-dependent individuals. *Journal of Consulting and Clinical Psychology* 66(3):541–548, 1998.

Stahler, G.J.; Shipley, T.E.; Kirby, K.C.; Godboldte, C.; Kerwin, M.E; Shandler, I.; and Simons, L. Development and initial demonstration of a community-based intervention for homeless, cocaine-using, African-American women. *Journal of Substance Abuse Treatment* 28(2):171–179, 2005.

Motivational Enhancement Therapy (Alcohol, Marijuana, Nicotine)

Motivational Enhancement Therapy (MET) is a counseling approach that helps individuals resolve their ambivalence about engaging in treatment and stopping their drug use. This approach aims to evoke rapid and internally motivated change, rather than guide the patient stepwise through the recovery process.

This therapy consists of an initial assessment battery session, followed by two to four individual treatment sessions with a therapist. In the first treatment session, the therapist provides feedback to the initial assessment, stimulating discussion about personal substance use and eliciting self-motivational statements. Motivational interviewing principles are used to strengthen motivation and build a plan for change. Coping strategies for high-risk situations are suggested and discussed with the patient. In subsequent sessions, the therapist monitors change, reviews cessation strategies being used, and continues to encourage commitment to change or sustained abstinence. Patients sometimes are encouraged to bring a significant other to sessions.

Research on MET suggests that its effects depend on the type of drug used by participants and on the goal of the intervention. This approach has been used successfully with people addicted to alcohol to both improve their engagement in treatment and reduce their problem drinking. MET has also been used successfully with marijuana-dependent adults when combined with cognitive-behavioral therapy, constituting a more comprehensive treatment approach. The results of MET are mixed for people abusing other drugs (e.g., heroin, cocaine, nicotine) and for adolescents who tend to use multiple drugs. In general, MET seems to be more effective for engaging drug abusers in treatment than for producing changes in drug use.

Further Reading:

Baker, A.; Lewin, T.; Reichler, H.; Clancy, R.; Carr, V.; Garrett, R.; Sly, K.; Devir, H.; and Terry, M. Evaluation of a motivational interview for substance use with psychiatric in-patient services. *Addiction* 97(10):1329-1337, 2002.

Haug, N.A.; Svikis, D.S.; and Diclemente, C. Motivational enhancement therapy for nicotine dependence in methadone-maintained pregnant women. *Psychology of Addictive Behaviors* 18(3):289-292, 2004.

Marijuana Treatment Project Research Group. Brief treatments for cannabis dependence: Findings from a randomized multisite trial. *Journal of Consulting and Clinical Psychology* 72(3):455-466, 2004.

Miller, W.R.; Yahne, C.E.; and Tonigan, J.S. Motivational interviewing in drug abuse services: A randomized trial. *Journal of Consulting and Clinical Psychology* 71(4):754-763, 2003.

Stotts, A.L.; Diclemente, C.C.; and Dolan-Mullen, P. One-to-one: A motivational intervention for resistant pregnant smokers. *Addictive Behaviors* 27(2):275-292, 2002.

The Matrix Model (Stimulants)

The Matrix Model provides a framework for engaging stimulant (e.g., methamphetamine and cocaine) abusers in treatment and helping them achieve abstinence. Patients learn about issues critical to addiction and relapse, receive direction and support from a trained therapist, and become familiar with self-help programs. Patients are monitored for drug use through urine testing.

The therapist functions simultaneously as teacher and coach, fostering a positive, encouraging relationship with the patient and using that relationship to reinforce positive behavior change. The interaction between the therapist and the patient is authentic and direct but not confrontational or parental. Therapists are trained to conduct treatment sessions in a way that promotes the patient's self-esteem, dignity, and self-worth. A positive relationship between patient and therapist is critical to patient retention.

Treatment materials draw heavily on other tested treatment approaches and, thus, include elements of relapse prevention, family and group therapies, drug education, and self-help participation. Detailed treatment manuals contain worksheets for individual sessions; other components include family education groups, early recovery skills groups, relapse prevention groups, combined sessions, urine tests, 12-step programs, relapse analysis, and social support groups.

A number of studies have demonstrated that participants treated using the Matrix Model show statistically significant reductions in drug and alcohol use, improvements in psychological indicators, and reduced risky sexual behaviors associated with HIV transmission.

Further Reading:

Huber, A.; Ling, W.; Shoptaw, S.; Gulati, V.; Brethen, P.; and Rawson, R. Integrating treatments for methamphetamine abuse: A psychosocial perspective. *Journal of Addictive Diseases* 16(4):41-50, 1997.

Rawson, R.; Shoptaw, S.J.; Obert, J.L.; McCann, M.J.; Hasson, A.L.; Marinelli-Casey, P.J.; Brethen, P.R.; and Ling, W. An intensive outpatient approach for cocaine abuse: The Matrix model. *Journal of Substance Abuse Treatment* 12(2):117-127, 1995.

Rawson, R.A.; Huber, A.; McCann, M.; Shoptaw, S.; Farabee, D.; Reiber, C.; and Ling, W. A comparison of contingency management and cognitive-behavioral approaches during methadone maintenance treatment for cocaine dependence. *Archives of General Psychiatry* 59(9):817-824, 2002.

12-Step Facilitation Therapy (Alcohol, Stimulants, Opiates)

Twelve-step facilitation therapy is an active engagement strategy designed to increase the likelihood of a substance abuser becoming affiliated with and actively involved in 12-step self-help groups, thereby promoting abstinence. Three key ideas predominate: (1) acceptance, which includes the realization that drug addiction is a chronic, progressive disease over which one has no control, that life has become unmanageable because of drugs, that willpower alone is insufficient to overcome the problem, and that abstinence is the only alternative; (2) surrender, which involves giving oneself over to a higher power, accepting the fellowship and support structure of other recovering addicted individuals, and following the recovery activities laid out by the 12-step program; and (3) active involvement in 12-step meetings and related activities. While the efficacy of 12-step programs (and 12-step facilitation) in treating alcohol dependence has been established, the research on its usefulness for other forms of substance abuse is more preliminary, but the treatment appears promising for helping drug abusers sustain recovery.

Further Reading:

Carroll, K.M.; Nich, C.; Ball, S.A.; McCance, E.; Frankforter, T.L.; and Rounsaville, B.J. One-year follow-up of disulfiram and psychotherapy for cocaine-alcohol users: Sustained effects of treatment. *Addiction* 95(9):1335-1349, 2000.

Donovan D.M., and Wells E.A. "Tweaking 12-step": The potential role of 12-Step self-help group involvement in methamphetamine recovery. *Addiction* 102(Suppl. 1):121-129, 2007.

Project MATCH Research Group. Matching alcoholism treatments to client heterogeneity: Project MATCH posttreatment drinking outcomes. *Journal of Studies on Alcohol* 58(1)7-29, 1997.

Family Behavior Therapy

Family Behavior Therapy (FBT), which has demonstrated positive results in both adults and adolescents, is aimed at addressing not only substance use problems but other co-occurring problems as well, such as conduct disorders, child mistreatment, depression, family conflict, and unemployment. FBT combines behavioral contracting with contingency management.

FBT involves the patient along with at least one significant other such as a cohabiting partner or a parent (in the case of adolescents). Therapists seek to engage families in applying the behavioral strategies taught in sessions and in acquiring new skills to improve the home environment. Patients are encouraged to develop behavioral goals for preventing substance use and HIV infection, which are anchored to a contingency management system. Substance-abusing parents are prompted to set goals related to effective parenting behaviors. During each session, the behavioral goals are reviewed, with rewards provided by significant others when goals are accomplished. Patients participate in treatment planning, choosing specific interventions from a menu of evidence-based treatment options. In a series of comparisons involving adolescents with and without conduct disorder, FBT was found to be more effective than supportive counseling.

Further Reading:

Azrin, N.H.; Donohue, B.; Besalel, V.A.; Kogan, E.S.; and Acierno, R. Youth drug abuse treatment: a controlled outcome study. *Journal of Child and Adolescent Substance Abuse* 3:1–16, 1994.

Carroll, K.M.; and Onken, L.S. Behavioral therapies for drug abuse. *American Journal of Psychiatry* 168(8):1452–1460, 2005.

Donohue, B.; Azrin, N.; Allen, D.N.; Romero, V.; Hill, H.H.; Tracy, K.; Lapota, H.; Gorney, S.; Abdel-al, R.; Caldas, D.; Herdzik, K.; Bradshaw, K.; Valdez, R.; and Van Hasselt, V.B. Family Behavior Therapy for substance abuse: A review of its intervention components and applicability. *Behavior Modification* 33:495–519, 2009.

LaPota, H.B.; Donohue, B.; Warren, C. S.; and Allen, D.N. Integration of a Healthy Living curriculum within Family Behavior Therapy: A clinical case example in a woman with a history of domestic violence, child neglect, drug abuse, and obesity. *Journal of Family Violence* 26:227–234, 2011.

Behavioral Therapies Primarily for Adolescents

Drug-abusing and addicted adolescents have unique treatment needs. Research has shown that treatments designed for and tested in adult populations often need to be modified to be effective in adolescents. Family involvement is a particularly important component for interventions targeting youth. Below are examples of behavioral interventions that employ these principles and have shown efficacy for treating addiction in youth.

Multisystemic Therapy

Multisystemic Therapy (MST) addresses the factors associated with serious antisocial behavior in children and adolescents who abuse alcohol and other drugs. These factors include characteristics of the child or adolescent (e.g., favorable attitudes toward drug use), the family (poor discipline, family conflict, parental drug abuse), peers (positive attitudes toward drug use), school (dropout, poor performance), and neighborhood (criminal subculture). By participating in intensive treatment in natural environments (homes, schools, and neighborhood settings), most youths and families complete a full course of treatment. MST significantly reduces adolescent drug use during treatment and for at least 6 months after treatment. Fewer incarcerations and out-of-home juvenile placements offset the cost of providing this intensive service and maintaining the clinicians' low caseloads.

Further Reading:

Henggeler, S.W.; Clingempeel, W.G.; Brondino, M.J.; and Pickrel, S.G. Four-year follow-up of multisystemic therapy with substance-abusing and substance-dependent juvenile offenders. *Journal of the American Academy of Child and Adolescent Psychiatry* 41(7):868-874, 2002.

Henggeler, S.W.; Rowland, M.D.; Randall, J.; Ward, D.M.; Pickrel, S.G.; Cunningham, P.B.; Miller, S.L.; Edwards, J.; Zealberg, J.J.; Hand, L.D.; and Santos, A.B. Home-based multisystemic therapy as an alternative to the hospitalization of youths in psychiatric crisis: Clinical outcomes. *Journal of the American Academy of Child and Adolescent Psychiatry* 38(11):1331-1339, 1999.

Henggeler, S.W.; Halliday-Boykins, C.A.; Cunningham, P.B.; Randall, J.; Shapiro, S.B.; and Chapman, J.E. Juvenile drug court: Enhancing outcomes by integrating evidence-based treatments. *Journal of Consulting and Clinical Psychology* 74(1):42–54, 2006.

Henggeler, S.W.; Pickrel, S.G.; Brondino, M.J.; and Crouch, J.L. Eliminating (almost) treatment dropout of substance-abusing or dependent delinquents through home-based multisystemic therapy. *The American Journal of Psychiatry* 153(3):427–428, 1996.

Huey, S.J.; Henggeler, S.W.; Brondino, M.J.; and Pickrel, S.G. Mechanisms of change in multisystemic therapy: Reducing delinquent behavior through therapist adherence and improved family functioning. *Journal of Consulting and Clinical Psychology* 68(3):451–467, 2000.

Multidimensional Family Therapy

Multidimensional Family Therapy (MDFT) for adolescents is an outpatient, family-based treatment for teenagers who abuse alcohol or other drugs. MDFT views adolescent drug use in terms of a network of influences (individual, family, peer, community) and suggests that reducing unwanted behavior and increasing desirable behavior occur in multiple ways in different settings. Treatment includes individual and family sessions held in the clinic, in the home, or with family members at the family court, school, or other community locations.

During individual sessions, the therapist and adolescent work on important developmental tasks, such as developing decision-making, negotiation, and problem-solving skills. Teenagers acquire vocational skills and skills in communicating their thoughts and feelings to deal better with life stressors. Parallel sessions are held with family members. Parents examine their particular parenting styles, learning to distinguish influence from control and to have a positive and developmentally appropriate influence on their children.

Further Reading:

Dennis, M.; Godley, S.H.; Diamond, G.; Tims, F.M.; Babor, T.; Donaldson, J.; Liddle, H.; Titus, J.C.; Kaminer, Y.; Webb, C.; Hamilton, N.; and Funk, R. The Cannabis Youth Treatment (CYT) Study: Main findings from two randomized clinical trials. *Journal of Substance Abuse Treatment* 27(3):197-213, 2004.

Liddle, H.A.; Dakof, G.A.; Parker, K.; Diamond, G.S.; Barrett, K;, and Tejeda, M. Multidimensional family therapy for adolescent drug abuse: Results of a randomized clinical trial. *The American Journal of Drug and Alcohol Abuse* 27(4):651-688, 2001.

Liddle, H.A., and Hogue, A. Multidimensional family therapy for adolescent substance abuse. In E.F. Wagner and H.B. Waldron (eds.), *Innovations in Adolescent Substance Abuse Interventions.* London: Pergamon/Elsevier Science, pp. 227-261, 2001.

Liddle, H.A.; Rowe, C.L.; Dakof, G.A.; Ungaro, R.A.; and Henderson, C.E. Early intervention for adolescent substance abuse: Pretreatment to posttreatment outcomes of a randomized clinical trial comparing multidimensional family therapy and peer group treatment. *Journal of Psychoactive Drugs* 36(1):49-63, 2004.

Schmidt, S.E.; Liddle, H.A.; and Dakof, G.A. Effects of multidimensional family therapy: Relationship of changes in parenting practices to symptom reduction in adolescent substance abuse. *Journal of Family Psychology* 10(1):1-16, 1996.

Brief Strategic Family Therapy

Brief Strategic Family Therapy (BSFT) targets family interactions that are thought to maintain or exacerbate adolescent drug abuse and other co-occurring problem behaviors. Such problem behaviors include conduct problems at home and at school, oppositional behavior, delinquency, associating with antisocial peers, aggressive and violent behavior, and risky sexual behavior. BSFT is based on a family systems approach to treatment, in which family members' behaviors are assumed to be interdependent such that the symptoms of one member (the drug-abusing adolescent, for example) are indicative, at least in part, of what else is occurring in the family system. The role of the BSFT counselor is to identify the patterns of family interaction that are associated with the adolescent's behavior problems and to assist in changing those problem-maintaining family patterns. BSFT is meant to be a flexible approach that can be adapted to a broad range of family situations in various settings (mental health clinics, drug abuse treatment programs, other social service settings, and families' homes) and in various treatment modalities (as a primary outpatient intervention, in combination with residential or day treatment, and as an aftercare/continuing-care service following residential treatment).

Further Reading:

Coatsworth, J.D.; Santisteban, D.A.; McBride, C.K.; and Szapocznik, J. Brief Strategic Family Therapy versus community control: Engagement, retention, and an exploration of the moderating role of adolescent severity. *Family Process* 40(3):313-332, 2001.

Kurtines, W.M.; Murray, E.J.; and Laperriere, A. Efficacy of intervention for engaging youth and families into treatment and some variables that may contribute to differential effectiveness. *Journal of Family Psychology* 10(1):35–44, 1996.

Santisteban, D.A.; Coatsworth, J.D.; Perez-Vidal, A.; Mitrani, V.; Jean-Gilles, M.; and Szapocznik, J. Brief Structural/Strategic Family Therapy with African-American and Hispanic high-risk youth. *Journal of Community Psychology* 25(5):453-471, 1997.

Santisteban, D.A.; Suarez-Morales, L.; Robbins, M.S.; and Szapocznik, J. Brief strategic family therapy: Lessons learned in efficacy research and challenges to blending research and practice. *Family Process* 45(2):259-271, 2006.

Santisteban, D.A.; Szapocznik, J.; Perez-Vidal, A.; Mitrani, V.; Jean-Gilles, M.; and Szapocznik, J. Brief Structural/Strategic Family Therapy with African-American and Hispanic high-risk youth. *Journal of Community Psychology* 25(5):453–471, 1997.

Szapocznik, J., et al. Engaging adolescent drug abusers and their families in treatment: A strategic structural systems approach. *Journal of Consulting and Clinical Psychology* 56(4):552-557, 1988.

Functional Family Therapy

Functional Family Therapy (FFT) is another treatment based on a family systems approach, in which an adolescent's behavior problems are seen as being created or maintained by a family's dysfunctional interaction patterns. FFT aims to reduce problem behaviors by improving communication, problem-solving, conflict resolution, and parenting skills. The intervention always includes the adolescent and at least one family member in each session. Principal treatment tactics include (1) engaging families in the treatment process and enhancing their motivation for change and (2) bringing about changes in family members' behavior using contingency management techniques, communication and problem-solving, behavioral contracts, and other behavioral interventions.

Further Reading:

Waldron, H.B.; Slesnick, N.; Brody, J.L.; Turner, C.W.; and Peterson, T.R. Treatment outcomes for adolescent substance abuse at 4- and 7-month assessments. *Journal of Consulting and Clinical Psychology* 69:802–813, 2001.

Waldron, H.B.; Turner, C. W.; and Ozechowski, T. J. Profiles of drug use behavior change for adolescents in treatment. *Addictive Behaviors* 30:1775–1796, 2005.

Adolescent Community Reinforcement Approach and Assertive Continuing Care

The Adolescent Community Reinforcement Approach (A-CRA) is another comprehensive substance abuse treatment intervention that involves the adolescent and his or her family. It seeks to support the individual's recovery by increasing family, social, and educational/vocational reinforcers. After assessing the adolescent's needs and levels of functioning, the therapist chooses from among 17 A-CRA procedures to address problem-solving, coping, and communication skills and to encourage active participation in positive social and recreational activities. A-CRA skills training involves role-playing and behavioral rehearsal.

Assertive Continuing Care (ACC) is a home-based continuing-care approach to preventing relapse. Weekly home visits take place over a 12- to 14-week period after an adolescent is discharged from residential, intensive outpatient, or regular outpatient treatment. Using positive and negative reinforcement to shape behaviors, along with training in problem-solving and communication skills, ACC combines A-CRA and assertive case management services (e.g., use of a multidisciplinary team of professionals, round-the-clock coverage, assertive outreach) to help adolescents and their caregivers acquire the skills to engage in positive social activities.

Further Reading:

Dennis, M.; Godley, S.H.; Diamond, G.; Tims, F.M.; Babor, T.; Donaldson, J.; Liddle, H.; Titus, J.C.; Kamier, Y.; Webb, C.; Hamilton, N.; and Funk R. The Cannabis Youth Treatment (CYT) Study: Main findings from two randomized trials. *Journal of Substance Abuse Treatment* 27:197–213, 2004.

Godley, S.H.; Garner, B.R.; Passetti, L.L.; Funk, R.R.; Dennis, M.L.; and Godley, M.D. Adolescent outpatient treatment and continuing care: Main findings from a randomized clinical trial. *Drug and Alcohol Dependence* Jul 1;110 (1-2):44–54, 2010.

Godley, M.D.; Godley, S.H.; Dennis, M.L.; Funk, R.; and Passetti, L.L. Preliminary outcomes from the assertive continuing care experiment for adolescents discharged from residential treatment. *Journal of Substance Abuse Treatment* 23:21–32, 2002.

Resources

National Agencies

The National Institute on Drug Abuse (NIDA) leads the Nation in scientific research on the health aspects of drug abuse and addiction. It supports and conducts research across a broad range of disciplines, including genetics, functional neuroimaging, social neuroscience, prevention, medication and behavioral therapies, and health services. It then disseminates the results of that research to significantly improve prevention and treatment and to inform policy as it relates to drug abuse and addiction. Additional information is available at drugabuse.gov or by calling 301-443-1124.

National Institute on Alcohol Abuse and Alcoholism (NIAAA)

The National Institute on Alcohol Abuse and Alcoholism (NIAAA) provides leadership in the national effort to reduce alcohol-related problems by conducting and supporting research in a wide range of scientific areas, including genetics, neuroscience, epidemiology, health risks and benefits of alcohol consumption, prevention, and treatment; coordinating and collaborating with other research institutes and Federal programs on alcohol-related issues; collaborating with international, national, State, and local institutions, organizations, agencies, and programs engaged in alcohol-related work; and translating and disseminating research findings to healthcare providers, researchers, policymakers, and the public. Additional information is available at www.niaaa.nih.gov or by calling 301-443-3860.

National Institute of Mental Health (NIMH)

The mission of National Institute of Mental Health (NIMH) is to transform the understanding and treatment of mental illnesses through basic and clinical research, paving the way for prevention, recovery, and cure. In support of this mission, NIMH generates research and promotes research training to fulfill the following four objectives: (1) promote discovery in the brain and behavioral sciences to fuel research on the causes of mental disorders; (2) chart mental illness trajectories to determine when, where, and how to intervene; (3) develop new and better interventions that incorporate the diverse needs and circumstances of people with mental illnesses; and (4) strengthen the public health impact of NIMH-supported research. Additional information is available at nimh.nih.gov or by calling 301-443-4513.

Center for Substance Abuse Treatment (CSAT)

The Center for Substance Abuse Treatment (CSAT), a part of the Substance Abuse and Mental Health Services Administration (SAMHSA), is responsible for supporting treatment services through a block grant program, as well as disseminating findings to the field and promoting their adoption. CSAT also operates the 24-hour National Treatment Referral Hotline (1-800-662-HELP), which offers information and referral services to people seeking treatment programs and other assistance. CSAT publications are available through SAMHSA's Store (store.samhsa.gov). Additional information about CSAT can be found on SAMHSA's Web site at www.samhsa.gov/about-us/who-we-are/offices-centers/csat.

Selected NIDA Educational Resources on Drug Addiction Treatment

The following are available from the NIDA *DrugPubs* Research Dissemination Center, the National Technical Information Service (NTIS), or the Government Printing Office (GPO). To order, refer to the *DrugPubs* (877-NIDANIH [643-2644]), NTIS (1-800-553-6847), or GPO (202-512-1800) number provided with the resource description.

Blending products. NIDA's Blending Initiative—a joint venture with SAMHSA and its nationwide network of Addiction Technology Transfer Centers (ATTCs) —uses "Blending Teams" of community practitioners, SAMHSA trainers, and NIDA researchers to create products and devise strategic dissemination plans for them. Completed products include those that address the value of buprenorphine therapy and onsite rapid HIV testing in community treatment programs; strategies for treating prescription opioid dependence; and the need to enhance healthcare workers' proficiency in using tools such as the Addiction

Severity Index (ASI), motivational interviewing, and motivational incentives. For more information on Blending products, please visit NIDA's Web site at drugabuse.gov/blending-initiative.

Addiction Severity Index. Provides a structured clinical interview designed to collect information about substance use and functioning in life areas from adult clients seeking drug abuse treatment. For more information on using the ASI and to obtain copies of the most recent edition, please visit triweb.tresearch.org/index.php/tools/download-asiinstruments-manuals/.

Drugs, Brains, and Behavior: The Science of Addiction (Reprinted 2010). This publication provides an overview of the science behind the disease of addiction. Publication #NIH 10-5605. Available online at drugabuse.gov/publications/science-addiction.

Seeking Drug Abuse Treatment: Know What To Ask (2011). This lay-friendly publication offers guidance in seeking drug abuse treatment and lists five questions to ask when searching for a treatment program. NIDA Publication #12-7764. Available online at drugabuse.gov/publications/seeking-drug-abuse-treatment.

Principles of Drug Abuse Treatment for Criminal Justice Populations: A Research-Based Guide (Revised 2012). Provides 13 essential treatment principles and includes resource information and answers to frequently asked questions. NIH Publication No.: 11-5316. Available online at drugabuse.gov/publications/principles-drug-abuse-treatment-criminal-justice-populations-research-based-guide.

NIDA *DrugFacts:* Treatment Approaches for Drug Addiction (Revised 2009). This is a fact sheet covering research findings on effective treatment approaches for drug abuse and addiction. Available online at drugabuse.gov/publications/drugfacts/treatment-approaches-drugaddiction.

Alcohol Alert **(published by NIAAA)**. This is a quarterly bulletin that disseminates important research findings on alcohol abuse and alcoholism. Available online at www.niaaa.nih.gov/publications/journals-and-reports/alcohol-alert.

Helping Patients Who Drink Too Much: A Clinicians's guide (published by NIAAA). This booklet is written for primary care and mental health clinicians and provides guidance in screening and managing alcohol-dependent patients. Available online at pubs.niaaa.nih.gov/publications/Practitioner/CliniciansGuide2005/clinicians_guide.htm.

Research Report **Series: Therapeutic Community** (2002). This report provides information on the role of residential drug-free settings and their role in the treatment process. NIH Publication #02-4877. Available online at drugabuse.gov/publications/research-reports/therapeutic-community.

Initiatives Designed to Move Treatment Research into Practice

Clinical Trials Network

Assessing the real-world effectiveness of evidence-based treatments is a crucial step in bringing research to practice. Established in 1999, NIDA's National Drug Abuse Treatment Clinical Trials Network (CTN) uses community settings with diverse patient populations and conditions to adjust and test protocols to meet the practical needs of addiction treatment. Since its inception, the CTN has tested pharmacological and behavioral interventions for drug abuse and addiction, along with common co-occurring conditions (e.g., HIV and PTSD) among various target populations, including adolescent drug abusers, pregnant drug-abusing women, and Spanish-speaking patients. The CTN has also tested prevention strategies in drug-abusing groups at high risk for HCV and HIV and has become a key element of NIDA's multipronged approach to move promising science-based drug addiction treatments rapidly into community settings. For more information on the CTN, please visit drugabuse.gov/CTN.

Criminal Justice-Drug Abuse Treatment Studies

NIDA is taking an approach similar to the CTN to enhance treatment for drug-addicted individuals involved with the criminal justice system through Criminal Justice–Drug Abuse Treatment Studies (CJ-DATS). Whereas NIDA's CTN has as its overriding mission the improvement of the quality of drug abuse treatment by moving innovative approaches into the larger community, research supported through CJ-DATS is designed to effect change by bringing new treatment models into the criminal justice system and thereby improve outcomes for offenders with substance use disorders. It seeks to achieve better integration of drug abuse treatment with other public health and public safety forums and represents a collaboration among NIDA; SAMHSA; the Centers for Disease Control and Prevention (CDC); Department of Justice agencies; and a host of drug treatment, criminal justice, and health and social service professionals.

Blending Teams

Another way in which NIDA is seeking to actively move science into practice is through a joint venture with SAMHSA and its nationwide network of Addiction Technology Transfer Centers (ATTCs). This process involves the collaborative efforts of community treatment practitioners, SAMHSA trainers, and NIDA researchers, some of whom form "Blending Teams" to create products and devise strategic dissemination plans for them. Through the creation of products designed to foster adoption of new treatment strategies, Blending Teams are instrumental in getting the latest evidence-based tools and practices into the hands of treatment professionals. To date, a number of products have been completed. Topics have included increasing awareness of the value of buprenorphine therapy and enhancing healthcare workers' proficiency in using tools such as the ASI, motivational interviewing, and motivational incentives. For more information on Blending products, please visit NIDA's Web site at drugabuse.gov/nidasamhsa-blending-initiative.

Other Federal Resources

NIDA *DrugPubs* Research Dissemination Center. NIDA publications and treatment materials are available from this information source. Staff provide assistance in English and Spanish, and have TTY/TDD capability. Phone: 877-NIDA-NIH (877-643-2644); TTY/TDD: 240-645-0228; fax: 240-645-0227; e-mail: drugpubs@nida.nih.gov; Web site: drugpubs.drugabuse.gov.

The National Registry of Evidence-Based Programs and Practices. This database of interventions for the prevention and treatment of mental and substance use disorders is maintained by SAMHSA and can be accessed at nrepp.samhsa.gov.

SAMHSA's Store has a wide range of products, including manuals, brochures, videos, and other publications. Phone: 800-487-4889; Web site: store.samhsa.gov.

The National Institute of Justice. As the research agency of the Department of Justice, the National Institute of Justice (NIJ) supports research, evaluation, and demonstration programs relating to drug abuse in the context of crime and the criminal justice system. For information, including a wealth of publications, contact the National Criminal Justice Reference Service at 800-851-3420 or 301-519-5500; or visit nij.gov.

Clinical Trials. For more information on federally and privately supported clinical trials, please visit clinicaltrials.gov.

This publication is available for your use and may be reproduced **in its entirety** without permission from the NIDA. Citation of the source is appreciated, using the following language: Source: National Institute on Drug Abuse; National Institutes of Health; U.S. Department of Health and Human Services.

Acknowledgments

The National Institute on Drug Abuse wishes to thank the following individuals for reviewing this publication.

Martin W. Adler, Ph.D.
Temple University School of Medicine

Kathleen Brady, M.D., Ph.D.
Medical University of South Carolina

Greg Brigham, Ph.D.
Maryhaven, Inc.

Kathleen M. Carroll, Ph.D.
Yale University School of Medicine

Richard R. Clayton, Ph.D.
University of Kentucky

Linda B. Cottler, Ph.D.
Washington University School of Medicine

David P. Friedman, Ph.D.
Wake Forest University
Bowman Gray School of Medicine

Reese T. Jones, M.D.
University of California at San Francisco

Nancy K. Mello, Ph.D.
Harvard Medical School

William R. Miller, Ph.D.
University of New Mexico

Charles P. O'Brien, M.D., Ph.D.
University of Pennsylvania

Jeffrey Selzer, M.D.
Zucker Hillside Hospital

Eric J. Simon, Ph.D.
New York University
Langone Medical Center

Jose Szapocznik, Ph.D.
University of Miami
Miller School of Medicine

George Woody, M.D.
University of Pennsylvania